Recent Results in Cancer Research 144

Springer
Berlin
Heidelberg
New York
Barcelona
Budapest
Hong Kong
London
Milan
Paris
Santa Clara
Singapore
Tokyo

R. Haas R. Kronenwett
G. Sczakiel (Eds.)

Advances in Hematopoietic Stem Cell Transplantation and Molecular Therapy

With 47 Figures and 8 Tables

Springer

Priv.-Doz. Dr. med. Rainer Haas
Dr. med. Ralf Kronenwett

Deutsches Krebsforschungszentrum
Klinische Kooperationseinheit
Molekulare Hämatologie/Onkologie (460)
Im Neuenheimer Feld 280
D-69120 Heidelberg

Priv.-Doz. Dr. rer. nat. Georg Sczakiel

Deutsches Krebsforschungszentrum
Forschungsschwerpunkt Angewandte
Tumorvirologie
Im Neuenheimer Feld 242
D-69120 Heidelberg

ISBN-13:978-3-642-46838-4 e-ISBN-13:978-3-642-46836-0
DOI: 10.1007/978-3-642-46836-0

Library of Congress Cataloging-in-Publication Data applied for
Die Deutsche Bibliothek – CIP-Einheitsaufnahme
Advances in hematopoietic stem cell transplantation and molecular therapy: with 8 tables / R. Haas ... (ed.). – Berlin; Heidelberg; New York; Barcelona; Budapest; Hong Kong; London; Milan; Paris; Santa Clara; Singapore; Tokyo: Springer, 1997
(Recent results in cancer research; Vol. 144)

Softcover reprint of the hardcover 1st edition 1998

Typesetting: K+V Fotosatz, Beerfelden

SPIN 10558982 19/3133-5 4 3 2 1 0 – Printed on acid-free paper

Preface

In 1985 when the first peripheral blood stem cell transplantation was carried out in Heidelberg one could not foresee the success of this therapeutic principle. Today, it is an established therapeutic option in the treatment of human diseases. In the interim, molecular therapeutic approaches such as the application of antibodies or gene therapy have become promising alternatives to the classical treatment of cancer. In 1995, the Clinical Cooperation Unit Molecular Hematology/Oncology was founded at the German Cancer Research Center to combine experience in clinical hematology and oncology and advances in basic research. To date several cooperative projects have been started which aim to facilitate the transfer of new developments in basic sciences to clinical applications. On September 13th and 14th 1996, an international symposium was held in Heidelberg at which clinical and basic scientists were invited to update and discuss the recent advances in hematopoietic stem cell transplantation and molecular therapy. The proceedings of this symposium are summarized in this book. Eighteen articles give an overview of the biology of hematopoietic stem cells, peripheral blood stem cell transplantation in patients with hematological malignancies, recent developments in molecular diagnosis, and gene therapeutic concepts. The symposium made transparent that successful future developments require cooperative research connecting basic science with clinical expertise.

We wish to thank the authors of the articles for their contributions and the publisher for support and cooperation.

Heidelberg, July 1997

R. Haas
R. Kronenwett
G. Sczakiel

Contents

List of Contributors*

Agape, P. [8]
Aicher, A. [70]
Barth, T. F. E. [53]
Bentz, M. [53]
Boiron, J. M. [8]
Brenner, M. K. [61]
Broustet, A. [8]
Brown, J. [46]
Buss, E. C. [93]
Cony-Makhoul, P. [8]
Döhner, H. [46, 53]
Engenhart, R. [27]
Fischer, K. [46]
Fruehauf, S. [93]
Fugazza, G. [46]
Gisselbrecht, C. [15]
Goldschmidt, H. [27]
Gückel, B. [78]
Günzburg, W. H. [116]
Haas, R. [1, 27, 86, 93, 127]
Hegenbart, U. [27]
Hehlmann, R. [36]
Hochhaus, A. [36]
Hohaus, S. [1, 27]
Hundsdoerfer, P. [93]
James, W. [139]
Karle, P. [116]
Klein, D. [116]
Kronenwett, R. [127]
Lichter, P. [46, 53]
Lindauer, M. [78]
Mahon, F. [8]
Marit, G. [8]
Meuer, S. C. [78]
Moebius, U. [78]
Mrochen, S. [116]
Murea, S. [1]
Ogniben, E. [86]
Pascheberg, U. [46]
Peter, W. [46]
Pezzutto, A. [70]
Pigneux, A. [8]
Plesch, A. [53]
Reichert, A. [36]
Reiffers, J. [8]
Reiter, A. [36]
Rudy, W. [78]
Saller, R. [116]
Salmons, B. [116]
Saußele, S. [36]
Scherer, S. W. [46]
Schramm, P. [46]
Skladny, H. [36]
Sparmann, G. [116]
Stewart, J. [46]
Stilgenbauer, S. [53]
Tsui, L.-C. [46]
Uckert, W. [116]

* The address of the principal author is given on the first page of each contribution.

[1] Page on which contribution begins.

Veldwijk, M.R.[93]
Voso, M.T.[1]
Wallmeier, M.[27]
Wannenmacher, M.[27]
Wermann, K.[93]
Werner, C.A.[53]
Westermann, J.[70]
Zeller, W.J.[93]

Mobilization and Selection of CD 34+ Cells

S. Hohaus, S. Murea, M. T. Voso and R. Haas

Department of Internal Medicine V, University of Heidelberg, Hospitalstraße 3, 69115 Heidelberg, Germany

High-risk patients with hematological malignancies and solid tumors may benefit from dose-escalated cytotoxic chemotherapy, provided that the tumor cells are chemosensitive as reflected by a dose-response relationship between the cytotoxic drugs administered and the degree of cell kill achieved. Since the first transplantation of peripheral blood stem cells (PBSC) in 1985, mobilized peripheral blood has gradually replaced the bone marrow as a source of hematopoietic stem cells (Körbling et al. 1986; Reiffers et al. 1986; Kessinger et al. 1988; see also Mahon et al., Gisselbrecht, and Goldschmidt et al., this volume). The faster hematological reconstitution after transplantation of PBSC compared to bone marrow ameliorates the dose-limiting myelotoxicity of high-dose regimens and results in a significant reduction of nonhematological toxicity (To et al. 1992; Schmitz et al. 1995). The use of hematopoietic growth factors is essential for efficient mobilization of PBSC (Haas et al. 1990; Hohaus et al. 1993; Haas and Murea 1995; Hohaus et al. 1997 a). In this setting, flow cytometry analysis with CD 34 staining permits counting of PBSC in a rapid and reliable fashion (Siena et al. 1991; Haas et al. 1994). It has become apparent that a minimum or threshold number of transplanted CD 34+ cells are needed for rapid and sustained hematological recovery (Hohaus et al. 1993; Haas et al. 1994; Schwartzberg et al. 1993; Weaver et al. 1995; Bensinger et al. 1993).

Additionally, blood-derived autografts contain fewer tumor cells than bone marrow in some malignancies such as breast cancer (Passos-Coelho et al. 1995; Ross et al. 1993). Further reduction of tumor cells in the transplant can be achieved using monoclonal antibodies for the purging of tumor cells or positive enrichment of CD 34+ cells (Berenson et al. 1991; Gorin et al. 1995; Hardwick et al. 1992). A purified population of CD 34+ cells is a sufficient autograft for the support of any high-dose therapy (Hohaus et al. 1977 b; Brugger et al. 1994). Improvement of mobilization conditions may help to provide blood-derived hematopoietic grafts with these characteristics.

Recent Results in Cancer Research, Vol. 144

Source of Hematopoietic Progenitor Cells: Bone Marrow Versus Mobilized Peripheral Blood

CD 34+ cells in bone marrow differ from their counterparts in mobilized peripheral blood with respect to both quantity and subset composition. In an intraindividual comparison of 208 cancer patients, the concentration of circulating CD 34+ cells in peripheral blood during G-CSF-stimulated marrow recovery after chemotherapy mobilization was 3.7-fold greater than in bone marrow before the start of mobilization (Hohaus et al. 1977 a). Differences in the composition of the CD 34+ cell population between these two sources were found by the expression of differentiation markers indicating lineage commitment: Thy-1 is found on early hematopoietic progenitor cells, and a greater proportion of G-CSF-mobilized CD 34+ cells than of bone marrow-derived CD 34+ cells express this molecule (Haas et al. 1995; Donahue et al. 1996). On the other hand, differentiation antigens such as CD 45 RA, representative of the late myeloid lineage, and CD 19, representative of the B-lymphoid lineage, are less expressed on CD 34+ cells mobilized by G-CSF-supported chemotherapy than on CD 34+ cells obtained from bone marrow during steady-state hematopoiesis (Haas et al. 1995; Dercksen et al. 1995). These data indicate that mobilized peripheral blood is a better source of hematopoietic progenitors enriched with a more primitive progenitor population, including true stem cells with high self-renewal ability.

Mobilization Regimen

The mobilization modality determines the efficiency of PBSC harvesting. In an intraindividual comparison of 17 patients with breast cancer and multiple myeloma, the yield of CD 34+ cells per leukapheresis after G-CSF-supported chemotherapy was 7-fold greater than after steady-state administration of G-CSF (Hohaus et al. 1997 a). In general, we treat patients with disease appropriate chemotherapy regimen followed by G-CSF in an attempt to combine effective antitumor therapy with mobilization of PBSC. The chemotherapy regimen for patients with breast cancer consists of either ifosfamide (7.5 g/m^2) and epirubicin (120 mg/m^2; IE) or paclitaxel (135 mg/m^2), ifosfamide (6 g/m^2), and epirubicin (90 mg/m^2; TIE), given over 3 days. Both regimens are effective for PBSC mobilization. The yield of CD 34+ cells after IE was 7.9±6.4/kg per leukapheresis in 41 patients, while TIE resulted in the harvest of 8.1±4.7/kg CD 34+ cells per leukapheresis in 15 patients.

Influence of Patient Characteristics on Mobilization Efficiency

Cytotoxic treatment impairs subsequent PBSC mobilization. In a group of 61 patients with hematological malignancies we found that each cycle of chemotherapy resulted in a decrease of 0.2×10^6 CD 34+ cells/kg per leukapheresis in nonirradiated patients, while large-field radiotherapy additionally reduced the collection efficiency by an average of 1.8×10^6/kg CD34+ cells (Haas et al. 1994). In 10 patients with advanced breast cancer, PBSC were harvested after the first and second cycles of IE therapy (Haas et al. 1977). The number of CD34+ cells/kg collected per leukapheresis was reduced 2.2-fold after the second cycle. PBSC harvesting is therefore most efficient before significant amounts of cytotoxic therapy have been administered.

Large-Volume Leukapheresis

The yield of PBSC can be increased by apheresis of 20 l peripheral blood instead of 10 l, a procedure generally termed "large-volume leukapheresis." Comparing 154 large-volume leukaphereses performed in 88 patients with 838 regular leukaphereses performed in 270 patients, the number of CD34+ cells harvested was 2.2-fold greater in the products of large-volume leukapheresis (Murea et al. 1996). This effect probably results from mobilization of CD34+ cells into peripheral blood during large-volume leukapheresis after 12–16 l blood have been processed. Using large-volume leukapheresis, the proportion of leukaphereses sufficient to support one high-dose cycle ($>2.5\times10^6$/kg CD34+ cells) was increased to 74%, compared to 52% of regular leukaphereses (Murea et al. 1996). For this reason we use products from large-volume apheresis when CD34+ cell enrichment is envisaged.

Tumor Cell Contamination

In patients with breast cancer, blood-derived autografts appear to be less contaminated with tumor cells than does bone marrow (Passos-Coelho et al. 1995; Ross et al. 1993). Isolated tumor cells in leukapheresis products can be detected by immunocytological staining with antibodies against epithelial antigens such as surface glycoproteins or intracytoplasmic cytokeratin (CK) filaments (Passos-Coelho et al. 1995; Ross et al. 1993; Diel et al. 1992). Using the monoclonal antibody CK18 as a marker for epithelial cells, 3 of 26 leukapheresis products (13.2%) harvested from patients following the first cycle of cytotoxic chemotherapy with IE were found to contain tumor cells. In contrast, only 2 of 62 leukapheresis products harvested after the second cycle of IE contained CK18+ cells (Haas et al. 1997). There was no difference in the proportion of tumor cells in leukapheresis products from patients with metastatic disease without bone and bone marrow metastases and those with primary breast cancer. The decrease in the number of leukapheresis products containing isolated tumor cells following the second cycle reflects the antitumor efficiency of the chemotherapy; however, the efficiency of collection of PBSC also decreased.

Large-Scale Selection of CD34+ Cells by Immunomagnetic Beads

In 25 patients with breast cancer, CD34+ cells from one of the patients' leukapheresis products were enriched using the Isolex 300 SA system, which is based on an immunomagnetic method (Baxter Immunotherapy, Irvine, CA). Six patients received the IE regimen and 19 patients the TIE regimen. Large-volume leukapheresis was performed after G-CSF-supported induction chemotherapy to harvest as many CD34+ cells as possible. On the basis of a good correlation between CD34+ cells in peripheral blood and the yield of CD34+ cells in the leukapheresis product, 26 large-volume leukaphereses which appeared to be sufficient for enrichment were selected (Fig. 1). The cells were incubated with the CD34 antibody 9C5. After binding to paramagnetic beads coated with sheep antimouse IgG1, the CD34+ cells were retained by a strong magnetic field, while the unbound cells were eluted. The CD34+ cells were released by cleavage of the CD34 epitope using chymopapain. The proportion of CD34+ cells before selection varied between 0.21% and 3.12%, corresponding to a number between 1.7×10^6 and 32.9×10^6/kg CD34+ cells. The selection procedure resulted in a highly purified CD34+ cell population (median 95%, range 82%–99%; Fig. 2). The recovery of CD34+ cells varied between 27% and 132% (median 80%). Despite a relatively greater loss of CD34+ cells with higher preselection numbers of mononuclear and CD34+ cells, there was good correlation between the starting number of CD34+ cells and the number recovered (Fig. 3). In total, 16 of 26 selection procedures resulted in numbers of CD34+ cell sufficient for at least two high-dose cycles.

Probing for tumor cells was performed using an immunocytological method as developed by S. Kaul (Department of Gynecology, University of Heidelberg). A cocktail of four monoclonal antibodies, including antibodies against breast mucin BM7 and BM8, the glycoprotein HEA, and the cytokeratin component 8, 18, 19, was used for an alkaline phosphatase-anti-alkaline phosphatase

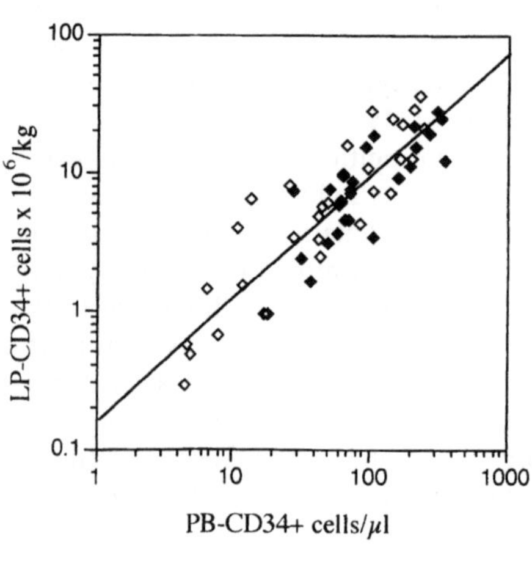

Fig. 1. Correlation between the number of CD34+ cells/μl peripheral blood (PB) and the yield of CD34+ cells in the leukapheresis products (LP) of the same day in 25 patients with breast cancer. The regression coefficient is 0.81. Twenty-six leukapheresis products – represented by *closed diamonds* – were chosen for immunomagnetic selection of CD34+ cells

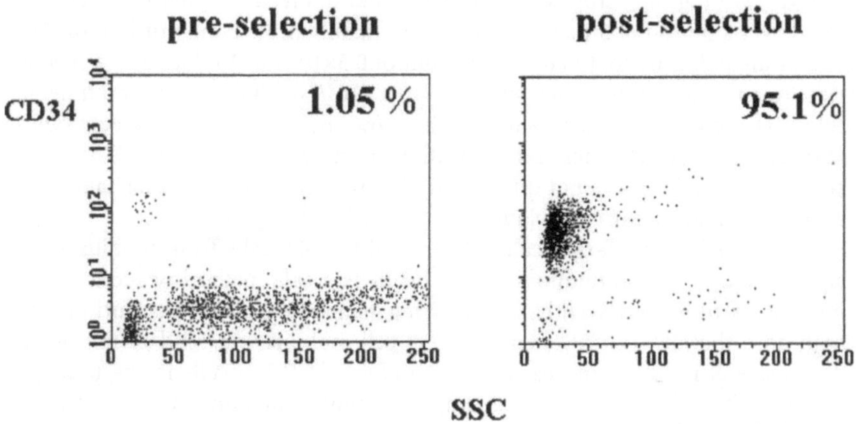

Fig. 2. Purity of CD 34+ cells before and after immunomagnetic selection using the Isolex 300 SA device for a representative patient. *SCC*, Sideward scatter

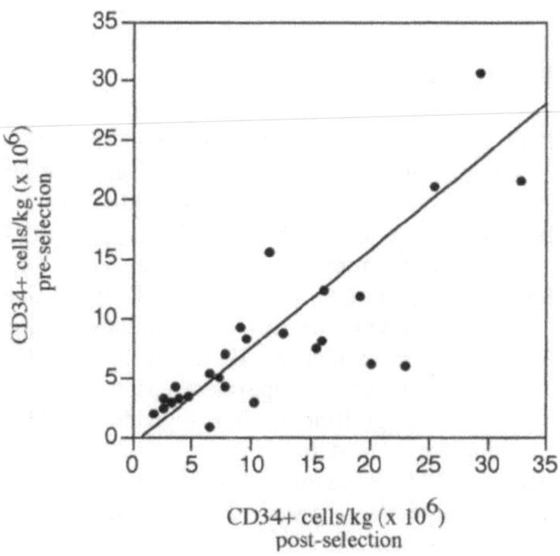

Fig. 3. Recovery of CD 34+ cells after immunomagnetic selection. The regression coefficient between the number of CD 34+ cells before and after selection is 0.82

(APAAP)-based method, permitting the detection of 1 tumor cell among 4×10^6 mononuclear cells (MNC). In 5 of 19 leukapheresis products, tumor cells were found at a concentration between 1 and 2 tumor cells per 10^6 MNC, whereas the selected CD 34+ cell fraction was free of tumor cells.

Transplantation of Selected CD 34+ Cells

A total of 40 high-dose cycles were supported using CD 34+ cells. High-dose therapy consisted of ifosfamide (12 g/m^2), epirubicin (180 mg/m^2), and carboplatin (900 mg/m^2), administered over a period of 5 days (24 cycles), or of paclitaxel (175 mg/m^2), etoposide (1500/m^2), and thiotepa (600 mg/m^2), administered over a period of 3 days (16 cycles). Hematological reconstitution was fast, with a median time to a neutrophil count of 0.5×10^9/l of 10 days and a median time to an unsubstituted platelet count of 20×10^9/l of 14 days. The rapid hematological recovery was associated with a low incidence of nonhematological toxicity. The hematological reconstitution in these patients after CD34+ cell-selected transplants was not different to that in a group of 75 breast cancer patients who underwent transplantation of unseparated products.

In conclusion, the large-scale selection of CD34+ cells from mobilized peripheral blood with immunomagnetic beads is a safe method of reducing the number of tumor cells without impairing hematological reconstitution after high-dose therapy. Improvement of stem cell mobilization renders the procedure more efficient by increasing the number of CD34+ cells in the products to start with. The impact of reducing the number of tumor cells on the relapse-free survival of patients is unclear at the moment, although some data indicate that tumor cells from the autograft may contribute to disease recurrence, as shown for patients with acute myeloid leukemia and neuroblastoma (Brenner et al. 1993).

References

Bensinger W, Singer J, Appelbaum F et al (1993) Autologous transplantation with peripheral blood mononuclear cells collected after administration of recombinant granulocyte colony-stimulating factor. Blood 81:3158–3163

Berenson RJ, Bensinger WI, Hill RS et al (1991) Engraftment after infusion of CD34+ marrow cells in patients with breast cancer or neuroblastoma. Blood 77:1717–1722

Brenner MK, Rill DR, Moen RC et al (1993) Gene marking to trace origin of relapse after autologous bone marrow transplantation. Lancet 341:85–86

Brugger W, Henschler R, Heimfeld S et al (1994) Positively selected autologous blood CD34+ cells and unseparated peripheral blood progenitor cells mediate identical hematopoietic engraftment after high-dose VP16, ifosfamide, carboplatin, and epirubicin. Blood 84:1421–1426

Dercksen MW, Rodenhuis S, Dirkson MKA et al (1995) Subsets of CD34+ cells and rapid hematopoietic recovery after peripheral-blood stem-cell transplantation. J Clin Oncol 13:1922–1932

Diel IJ, Kaufmann M, Goerner R et al (1992) Detection of tumor cells in bone marrow of patients with primary breast cancer: a prognostic factor for distant metastasis. J Clin Oncol 10:1534–1539

Donahue RE, Kirby MR, Metzger ME et al (1996) Peripheral blood CD34+ cells differ from bone marrow CD34+ cells in Thy-1 expression and cell cycle status in nonhuman primates mobilized or not mobilized with granulocyte-stimulating factor and/or stem cell factor. Blood 87:1644–1653

Gorin NC, Lopez M, Laporte JP et al (1995) Preparation and successful engraftment of purified CD34+ bone marrow progenitor cells in patients with non-Hodgkin's lymphoma. Blood 85:1647–1654

Haas R, Murea S (1995) The role of granulocyte colony-stimulating factor in mobilization and transplantation of peripheral blood progenitor and stem cells. Cytokines Mol Ther 1:249–270

Haas R, Ho AD, Bredthauer U et al (1990) Successful autologous transplantation of blood stem cells mobilized with recombinant human granulocyte-macrophage colony-stimulating factor. Exp Hematol 18:94–98

Haas R, Möhle R, Frühauf S et al (1994) Patient characteristics associated with successful mobilizing and autografting of peripheral blood progenitor cells in malignant lymphoma. Blood 83:3787–3794

Haas R, Möhle R, Pförsich M et al (1995) Blood-derived autografts collected during granulocyte colony-stimulating factor-enhanced recovery are enriched with early Thy-1+ hematopoietic progenitor cells. Blood 85:1936–1943

Haas R, Schmid H, Hahn U et al (1997) Tandem high-dose therapy with ifosfamide, epirubicin, carboplatin and peripheral blood stem cell support is an effective adjuvant treatment for high-risk primary breast cancer. Eur J Cancer (in press)

Hardwick RA, Kulcinski D, Mansour V et al (1992) Design of large-scale separation systems for positive and negative immunomagnetic selection of cells using super-paramagnetic microspheres. J Hematother 1:379–386

Hohaus S, Goldschmidt H, Ehrhardt R, Haas R (1993) Successful autografting following myeloablative conditioning therapy with blood stem cells mobilized by chemotherapy plus rhG-CSF. Exp Hematol 21:508–514

Hohaus S, Voso MT, Haas R (1997a) The role of cytokines for the mobilization of blood stem cells. In: Reiffers J, Goldman R, Armitage J (eds) Blood stem cell transplantation. Martin Dunitz, London (in press)

Hohaus S, Pförsich M, Murea S et al (1997b) Immunomagnetic selection of CD 34+ peripheral blood stem cells for autografting in patients with breast cancer. Br J Haematol (in press)

Kessinger A, Armitage JO, Landmark JD et al (1988) Autologous peripheral hematopoietic stem cell transplantation restores hamatopoietic function following marrow ablative therapy. Blood 71:723–727

Körbling M, Dörken B, Ho AD et al (1986) Autologous transplantation of blood-derived hemopoietic stem cells after myeloablative therapy in a patient with Burkitt's lymphoma. Blood 67:529–532

Murea S, Goldschmidt H, Hahn U et al (1996) Successful collection and transplantation of peripheral blood stem cells in cancer patients using large-volume leukaphereses. J Clin Apheresis 11:185–194

Passos-Coelho JL, Ross AA, Moss TJ et al (1995) Absence of breast cancer cells in a single-day peripheral blood progenitor cell collection after priming with cyclophosphamide and granulocyte-macrophage colony-stimulating factor. Blood 85:1138–1143

Reiffers J, Bernard P, David B et al (1986) Successful autologous transplantation with peripheral blood hemopoietic cells in a patient with acute leukemia. Exp Hematol 14:312–315

Ross AA, Cooper BW, Lazarus HM et al (1993) Detection and viability of tumor cells in peripheral blood stem cell collections from breast cancer patients using immunocytochemical and clonogenic assay techniques. Blood 82:2605–2610

Schmitz N, Dreger P, Suttorp M et al (1995) Primary transplantation of allogeneic peripheral blood progenitor cells mobilized by filgrastim (granulocyte colony-stimulating factor). Blood 85:1666–1672

Schwartzberg L, Birch R, Blanco R et al (1993) Rapid and sustained hematopoietic reconstitution by peripheral blood stem cell infusion alone following high-dose chemotherapy. Bone Marrow Transplant 11:369–374

Siena A, Bregni M, Brando B et al (1991) Flow cytometry for clinical estimation of circulating hematopoietic progenitors for autologous transplantation in cancer patients. Blood 77:400–409

To LB, Roberts MM, Haylock DN et al (1992) Comparison of haematological recovery times and supportive care requirements of autologous recovery phase peripheral blood stem cell transplants, autologous bone marrow transplants and allogeneic bone marrow transplants. Bone Marrow Transplant 9:277–284

Weaver CH, Hazelton B, Birch R et al (1995) An analysis of engraftment kinetics as a function of the CD 34 content of peripheral blood progenitor cell collections in 692 patients after the administration of myeloablative chemotherapy. Blood 86:3961–3969

Autologous Stem Cell Transplantation for Chronic Myeloid Leukemia

F.X. Mahon, G. Marit, J.M. Boiron, P. Cony-Makhoul, P. Agape, A. Pigneux, A. Broustet, and J. Reiffers

Department of Hematology, Haut-Lévêque Hospital, CHU Bordeaux, 33604 Pessac, France

Introduction

Autologous stem cell transplantation (ASCT) has been used in chronic myeloid leukemia (CML) for the past 20 years. ASCT was first proposed in CML in transformation with the objective of achieving a second chronic phase lasting, hopefully, as long as the initial chronic phase. Despite the use of various myeloablative conditioning regimens, however, including either total body irradiation or busulfan (14–16 mg/kg), this objective was not achieved, as patients usually develop a recurrent blastic transformation within 3–6 months after ASCT. Given these disappointing results, the use of ASCT was abandoned in this indication in the early 1980s.

ASCT undertaken in CML patients in blast crisis was essentially performed using hematopoietic blood stem cells obtained by leukapheresis at the time of initial diagnosis. Several authors, notably Goldman et al. (1978), have demonstrated that peripheral blood stem cells contain a high proportion of hematopoietic progenitor cells (as many CFU-GM in one leukapheresis as in a medullary harvest). Since the karyotype of cells obtained by leukapheresis showed the presence of Philadelphia chromosome (ph)-positive metaphases, certain hematopoietic reconstitutions were also done using stem cells derived from a normal hematopoietic source, probably having a proliferative advantage over leukemic progenitors (Reiffers et al. 1983). These observations were made at about the same period as for the first time, Coulombel et al. (1983) demonstrated the presence of normal (Ph-negative) hematopoietic progenitor cells in the marrow of patients with CML. Since these observations were made, the presence of normal hematopoietic cells has also been confirmed not only in the marrow (Verfaillie et al. 1992) but also in peripheral blood (Petzer et al. 1996). These normal progenitor cells were essentially shown to belong to a subfraction of very immature CD34-positive cells (CD34+ CD38- or CD34+ DR- or Thy-1+) which according to our experience (Jazwiec et al. 1995) are resistant to 5-fluorouracil.

The possibility of obtaining "cytogenetic conversions" led certain authors to propose ASCT in chronic-phase CML patients. However, this therapeutic alternative has not been extensively applied, as patients with an HLA identical donor and under 45 years of age usually benefit from an allogeneic bone marrow transplant, while all other patients receive therapy with recombinant interferon-α (IFN). However, in the last few years, some data have suggested that ASCT can prolong survival in CML patients. We summarize these data here and discuss under what conditions ASCT might be used as a therapeutic alternative for the next decade.

ASCT in Chronic Phase CML: Main Results to Date

The main results of ASCT in chronic phase CML have been obtained in Europe in London, Rome, and Bordeaux, and in North America by the Vancouver, Houston, and Minneapolis groups. The results obtained by these various groups are similar (Haines et al. 1984; Meloni et al. 1990; Reiffers et al. 1993a; Barnett et al. 1994; Khourie et al. 1996; McGlave et al. 1990). The most encouraging result is that ASCT has little toxicity; hematopoietic reconstitution using peripheral blood stem cells is usually rapid (less than 15 days) and a cytogenetic conversion, sometimes of very long duration and without any therapy after the transplantation, has been observed in 15–40% of the cases. Since most of the studies performed were pilot phase II trials, with a small number of patients included and a short follow-up time, it has never been demonstrated that ASCT can prolong survival. However, it has been reported that survival of patients who underwent ASCT at the Hammersmith Hospital (London group) was longer than that observed for patients receiving hydroxyurea or busulfan in the UK Medical Researach Council study (Hoyle et al. 1994). No study has ever compared ASCT with interferon-α.

Several retrospective analyses of ASCT results in chronic phase CML patients have been performed by cooperative groups: the France Auto Greffe group has analyzed results of 23 CML patients who underwent transplantation during chronic phase, but with adverse prognostic factors such as a high Sokal index at diagnosis or lack of response to interferon treatment (defined as absence of clinical response after 6 months or absence of cytogenetic response after 12 months of treatment). All such patients underwent transplantation of peripheral blood cells obtained at diagnosis, after a myeloablative treatment which included busulfan (4 mg/kg per day for 4 days) and melphalan (140 mg/m^2). The probability of survival of these 23 patients, at 3 years, was 68.8±23% (95% confidence interval) (Reiffers et al. 1993b).

In the cooperative study published by McGlave et al. (1994), in a sample of 200 patients undergoing transplantation in eight different European and American centers, the survival at 6 years in those transplanted during chronic phase was greater than 50%. No other prognostic factors apart from age had an impact on survival.

In the analysis of the European registry, 170 patients were studied. The overall results are identical to those of the above study, even though most patients had adverse prognostic factors such a Sokal index greater than 1.2 or a resistance to IFN (Reiffers et al. 1994). Utilizing the Houston criteria, the responses observed in these 170 patients were as follows: the actuarial percentage of complete hematological response at 5 years was in the range of 75%; the actuarial percentage of complete cytogenetic response at 24 months was in the range of 35% (the median duration of these responses has not been reached); the 5-year survival was 75%; and the most significant prognostic factor for survival was a major or complete response after ASCT. Since most of these transplant patients had adverse prognostic factors, this study suggests that ASCT may prolong survival. This benefit may be due to a decrease in overall tumor burden or to other ill-defined factors. In addition, it is now evident that in certain IFN-resistant patients, ASCT restores sensitivity to IFN.

Although these studies suggest that ASCT could improve survival, this suggestion could only be demonstrated by a multicenter prospective randomized trial, given the low incidence of CML. Such a trial has been initiated in France by the Société Française de Greffe de Moelle.

Future Perspectives

As discussed above, certain data suggest that ASCT can prolong the survival of patients with CML. In no case, however, can ASCT be seen as a cure for CML, at least for the next few years. Some authors believe that in order to benefit survival, ASCT must be followed by other treatment, such as with recombinant IFN-α.

Although it is believed that ASCT can prolong survival of CML patients in chronic phase, what the best transplant modality is is still unknown: there is no indication that one conditioning regimen is superior to any other, or that peripheral stem cells are superior to marrow-harvested stem cells (except for the hematologic reconstitution) or that ex vivo treatment of transplanted cells prior to reinfusion prolongs survival. However, since Deisseroth et al. (1994) reported that leukemic cells present in the stem cell harvest could contribute to disease relapse, some teams think it indispensible to use an ex vivo or in vivo purging technique for ASCT in CML patients (see Brenner, this volume).

Techniques for ex vivo purging of hematopoietic cells in CML are varied. They generally employ chemical agents (usually derivatives of cyclophosphamide or, more recently, of tyrosine kinase inhibitors), IFN-α or IFN-γ, bone marrow culture or antisense oligonucleotides (see Günzburg et al., this volume). None of these methods is superior to any other and, as discussed above, no survival advantage has been demonstrated compared to that observed with the use of nonmanipulated cells.

In the work performed by Brito-Babapulle et al. (1989), cytogenetic conversions, often of long duration (more than 3 years after transplant) without any other therapeutic interventions after ASCT, were observed in patients transplanted with peripheral stem cells harvested at initial diagnosis and containing only Ph-positive cells. Other cytogenetic conversions were also observed after ASCT using marrow or peripheral ex vivo treated cells, but these conversions did not appear to be more frequent or durable than those observed without ex vivo purging. In the work done by McGlave et al. (1990) in six patients transplanted with IFN-γ-treated marrow, complete cytogenetic conversion was noted in three patients, but was of short duration (never exceeding 12 months) in all three. In the recently published work of Barnett et al. (1994) in 22 patients, cytogenetic conversions were frequently observed using ex vivo cultured marrow (for 10–15 days), but these patients were selected on the basis of biological criteria and the median follow-up was of short duration (31 months). Results observed after treatment of marrow using derivatives of cyclophosphamide are no better and relate to only a few patients (Carlo-Stella et al. 1991). Results of ex vivo marrow manipulation using antisense oligonucleotides are still preliminary. All these ex vivo techniques are highly toxic to stem cells and could require a longer hematopoietic recuperation time after transplant (De Fabritiis et al. 1995).

Given the relative disappointment of these methods, many authors have recently focused their work on ASCT using cells harvested after several different in vivo treatments. This is not by any means a new therapeutic strategy, since approximately 10 years ago we administered intensive chemotherapy to ten patients in order to harvest Ph-negative bone marrow cells during the hematopoietic recovery (Reiffers et al. 1987). This approach was also undertaken in Italy in patients who had a complete or partial response after IFN-α treatment, but was disappointing because IFN-α, being profoundly hemotoxic, rendered a bone marrow with very few hematopoietic progenitor cells, which was not of much value for ASCT (Italian Cooperative Study Group on Chronic Myeloid Leukemia 1993).

Recently, along with the introduction of growth factors, it was demonstrated by the Genoa group (Carella et al. 1993) that, in patients in chronic phase, leukaphereses performed during the hematologic recovery period following intensive chemotherapy (ICE protocol: idarubicin+ara-C+etoposide) followed by G-CSF can contain up to 100% of normal metaphases. The same authors have demonstrated that the frequency with which it was possible to obtain normal metaphases in leukaphereses was inversely proportional to the duration of the chronic phase. When these leukaphereses were used for autologous transplant, they also observed that cytogenetic conversions were regularly obtained. These interesting results must be confirmed by other groups in order to evaluate the toxicity of the ICE chemotherapy protocol and the impact on survival of this new strategy of autologous transplant.

Another in vivo purging method is to administer only cytokines (without chemotherapy) in the hope of stimulating preferentially normal cells to be collected by leukapheresis. We have conducted a pilot study in which G-CSF (lenograstim 150 $\mu g/m^2$) was administered for 7–10 days to complete or partial cytogenetically responding patients (>65% normal mitoses) after IFN treatment (Reiffers et al. 1996). Even though as the dose of G-CSF was relatively low, recirculation of hematopoietic progenitor cells was satisfactory, allowing collection of a sufficient number of CFU-GM and CD34-positive cells in 22 out of 23 cases. In addition, in 12 patients, there was at least one leukapheresis with sufficient progenitor cells and total absence of Ph-positive cells. Some of these leukaphereses were found to be negative for the BCR-ABL transcript after amplification (see Hochhaus et al., this volume). Although performed in patients who were responding to IFN therapy (without a transplant indication), these leukaphereses have not yet been used for autologous transplant. Similar results, although preliminary, have been observed by others (Carreras et al. 1997; Archimbaud et al. 1996). It is noteworthy that in patients in partial response during IFN therapy, G-CSF can allow collection of exclusively Ph-negative cells, as if in these patients G-CSF had a preferential stimulatory effect on normal cells (Archimbaud et al. 1996). If this observation is confirmed, it may result in further exploration of new cytokine regimens.

Conclusion

Many data indicate that ASCT (or high-dose chemotherapy preceding the reinfusion of hematopoietic cells) can have a beneficial effect on survival in certain patients with CML. Since the toxicity of ASCT is low, this effect of ASCT needs to be further evaluated within the setting of a prospective multicenter trial. In view of the recent biologic data allowing the possible selection of normal cells in CML, the optimal conditions in which ASCT is to be performed could be further defined.

References

Archimbaud E, Michalet M, Philip I, Sebban C, Guilhot F, Fière D (1996) G-CSF (figrastim) added to interferon alpha to mobilize peripheral blood stem cells for autologous transplant in chronic myeloid leukemia. Bone Marrow Transplant 17 Suppl 1:S4

Barnett MJ, Eaves CJ, Phillips GL, Gascoyne RD, Hogge DE, Horsman DE, Humphries RK, Klingemann H-G, Lansdorp PM, Nantel SH, Reece DE, Shepherd JD, Spinelli JJ, Sutherland HJ, Eaves AC (1994) Autografting with cultured marrow in chronic myeloid leukemia:results of a pilot study. Blood 84:724–732

Brito-Babapulle F, Bowcock SJ, Marcus RE, Apperley J, Th'ng KH, Dowding C, Guo AP, Catowsky D, Galton DAG, Goldman JM (1989) Autografting for patients with chronic myeloid leukaemia in chronic phase: peripheral blood stem cells may have a finite capacity for maintaining haemopoiesis. Br J Haematol 73:76–81

Carella AM, Podesta M, Frassoni F, Raffo MR, Pollicardo N, Pungolino E, Vimercati R, Sessarego M, Parodi C, Rabitti C, Ferrero R, Benvenuto F, Figari O, Carlier P, Levcasic G, Valbonesi M, Vitale V, Giordano D, Pierluigi D, Nati S, Guerracio A, Rosso C, Saglio G (1993) Collection of normal blood repopulating cells during early hematopoietic recovery after intensive conventional chemotherapy in chronic myelogenous leukemia. Bone Marrow Transplant 12:267–271

Carlo-Stella C, Mangoni L, Piovani G, Almici C, Garau D, Caramatti C, Rizzoli V (1991) In vitro purging in chronic myelogenous leukemia: effect of mafosfamide and recombinant granulocyte-macrophage colony-stimulating factor. Bone Marrow Transplant 8:265–271

Carreras E, Sierra J, Rovira M, Urbano-Ispiza A, Martinez C, Nomdedeu B, Cervantes F, Marin P, Rozman C, Monserrat E (1997) Successful autografting in chronic myelogenous leukemia using Philadelphia negative blood progenitor cell mobilized with rHuG-GCF alone in a patient responding to alpha-interferon. Br J Haematol (in press)

Coulombel L, Kalousek DK, Eaves CJ, Gupta CM, Eaves AC (1983) Long-term marrow culture reveals chromosomally normal hematopoietic progenitor cells in patients with Philadelphia chromosome positive chronic myelogenous leukemia. N Engl J Med 308:1493–1498

De Fabritiis P, Amadori S, Petti MC, Mancini M, Montefusco E, Picardi A, Geiser T, Campbell K, Calabretta B, Mandelli F (1995) In vitro purging with BCR-ABL antisense oligonucleotides does not prevent haematologic reconstitution after autologous bone marrow transplantation. Leukemia 9:662–668

Deisseroth AB, Zu Z, Claxton D, Hanania EG, Fu S, Ellerson D, Goldberg L, Thomas M, Janicek K, Anderson WF, Hester J, Korbling M, Durett A, Moen R, Berenson R, Heimfeld S, Hamer J, Calvert L, Tibbits P, Talpaz M, Kantarjian H, Champlin R, Reading C (1994) Genetic marking shows that Ph+ cells present in autologous transplants of chronic myelogenous leukemia (CML) contribute to relapse after autologous bone marrow in CML. Blood 83:3068–3076

Goldman JM, Th'ng KH, Park DS, Spiers ASD, Lowenthal RM, Ruutu T (1978) Collection, cryopreservation and subsequent viability of haemopoietic stem cells intended for treatment of chronic granulocytic leukemia in blast-cell transformation. Br J Haematol 40:185–195

Haines ME, Goldman JM, Worsley AM, McCarthy DM, Wyatt SE, Dowding C, Kearny L, Th'ng KH, Wareham NJ, Pollock A, Galvin MC, Samson D, Geary CG, Catovsky D, Galton DAG (1984) Chemotherapy and autografting for chronic granulocytic leukemia in transformation: probable prolongation of survival in some patients. Br J Haematol 58:711–721

Hoyle C, Gray R, Goldman J (1994) Autografting for patients with CML in chronic phase: an update. Br J Haematol 86:76–81

Italian Cooperative Study Group (ICSG) on Chronic Myeloid Leukemia (1993) Karyotype conversion by interferon as preparative treatment for autologous BMT in Ph positive CML. Leuk Lymphoma 11 Suppl 1:277–280

Jazwiec B, Mahon FX, Pigneux A, Pigeonnier V, Reiffers J (1995) 5-Fluorouracil resistant CD34+ cell population from peripheral blood of CML patients contains Bcr-Abl negative progenitors cells. Exp Hematol 23:1509–1514

Khouri IF, Kantarjian H, Talpaz M, Giralt S, Rios MO, Hester JP, Champlin RE, Deisseroth AB (1996) Results with high-dose chemotherapy and unpurged autologous stem cell transplantation in 73 patients with chronic myelogenous leukemia: the MD Anderson experience. Bone Marrow Transplant 17:775–779

McGlave PB, Arthur D, Miller WJ, Lasky L, Kersey J (1990) Autologous transplantation for CML using marrow treated ex vivo with recombinant human interferon gamma. Bone Marrow Transplant 6:115–120

McGlave PB, De Fabritiis P, Deisseroth J, Goldman J, Barnett M, Reiffers J, Simonsson B, Carella A, Aeppli D (1994) Autologous transplants for chronic myelogenous leukemia: results from eight transplant groups. Lancet 343:1486–1488

Meloni G, de Fabritiis P, Alimena F, Malagnino F, Montefusco E, Sandrelli E, Pinto R, Vignetti M, Lo Coco F, Mandelli F (1990) Autologous bone marrow transplantation or peripheral blood stem cell transplantation for patients with chronic myelogenous leukemia in chronic phase. Bone Marrow Transplant 4 Suppl 14:92–94

Petzer AL, Eaves CJ, Lansdorp PM, Ponchio MJ, Barnett MJ, Eaves AC (1996) Characterization of primitive subpopulation of normal and leukemic cells in the blood of patients with newly diagnosed as well as established chronic myeloid leukemia. Blood 88:2162–2171

Reiffers J, Broustet A, Goldman JM (1983) Philadelphia chromosome negative progenitors in chronic granulocytic leukaemia. N Engl J Med 309:1460

Reiffers J, Maraninchi D, Marit G, Bertheas MF, Bernard P, Blaise D, David B, Lepeu G, Feuillatre F, Novakovitch G, Wen-Zong Qi, Gastaut JA, Broustet A, Carcassonne Y (1987) Autologous transplantation of Ph-positive cell depleted marrow in chronic granulocytic leukemia. In: Dicke K, Spitzer G, Jagannath S (eds) Autologous bone marrow transplantation. University of Texas MD Anderson Hospital and Tumor Institute, Houston, pp 199–203

Reiffers J, Montastruc M, Marit G, Cony-Makhoul P, Faberes C, Bilhou-Nabera C, Gharbi M, Bernard P, Vezon G, Broustet A (1993a) Autologous blood stem cell transplantation followed by recombinant alpha interferon as treatment for patients with high-risk chronic myelogenous leukemia: a report of 32 cases. Leuk Lymphoma 11 Suppl 1:297–299

Reiffers J, Cahn JY, Montastruc M, Caillot D, Souillet G, Leblond V, Troncy EJ, Faberes C (1993b) Peripheral blood stem cell transplantation followed by recombinant alpha interferon for chronic myelogeneous leukemia in chronic phase: preliminary results. Stem Cells 11:23–24

Reiffers J, Goldman J, Meloni G, Cahn JY, Gratwohl A on behalf of the Chronic Leukemia Working Party of the EBMT (1994) Autologous stem cell transplantation in chronic myelogenous leukemia: a retrospective analysis of the European Group for Bone Marrow Transplantation. Bone Marrow Transplant 14:407–410

Reiffers J, Taylor K, Gluckman E, Gorin N, Carrella A, Destrée D (1996) Ph negative blood progenitors cells can be successfully collected with lenogratim in patients with chronic myeloid leukemia good responders to alpha-interferon. Bone Marrow Transplant 17 Suppl 1:54

Verfaillie CM, Miller WJ, Boylan K, McGlave PB (1992) Selection of benign primitive hematopoietic progenitors in chronic myelogenous leukemia on the basis of HLA-DR antigen expression. Blood 79:1003–1005

Autologous Stem Cell Transplantation in Aggressive Non-Hodgkin's Lymphoma

C. Gisselbrecht

Institute of Hematology, Saint Louis Hospital, 1, avenue Claude Vellefaux, 75010 Paris, France

Abstract

High-dose therapy with autologous stem cell transplantation (ASCT) has been widely used in the past decade for treating aggressive non-Hodgkin's lymphoma in situations in which conventional therapy was not likely to cure patients. In patients achieving complete remission (CR), ASCT has been proposed for consolidation in a group of lymphoma patients sharing adverse prognostic factors with a high risk of relapse. Results from pilot studies were encouraging. Analysis of the large randomized LNH 87 trial showed an increased survival and disease-free survival advantage for ASCT performed after CR when compared to conventional chemotherapy if patients with two or more adverse factors were included. For patients who do not achieve CR after conventional treatment, but who are still sensitive to chemotherapy, ASCT may improve results. Pilot studies as well as randomized studies offer support for this approach. Intensive treatment with ASCT has been reported in thousands of relapsing lymphoma patients. For those remaining sensitive to salvage chemotherapy at 5 years, a 40% probability of disease-free survival has been uniformly noted. Moreover, these results were confirmed by the randomized PARMA study testing ASCT vs conventional chemotherapy. ASCT is accepted by most centers as the treatment of choice for relapsing lymphoma. For lymphoblastic lymphoma and Burkitt's lymphoma, the role of ASCT in first CR is not well defined, although results from pilot studies and the analysis of registry data support the use of ASCT in lymphoblastic lymphoma with adverse prognostic factors. In conclusion, data supporting the use of ASCT in lymphoma in different settings has been provided by numerous nonrandomized trials. Completed randomized studies clearly demonstrate a benefit for ASCT in most relapsing patients as well as a subset of patients with poor prognosis. The socioeconomic implications of such results must be evaluated, especially since the development of peripheral hematopoietic stem cells will reduce both toxicity and cost.

Recent Results in Cancer Research, Vol. 144

Introduction

In the past ten years, a considerable amount of effort has been devoted to evaluating whether intensive treatment will improve the outcome for patients with intermediate and high grade non-Hodgkin's lymphomas (NHL). Despite promising results in pilot studies testing second and third-generation therapies, several carefully conducted clinical trials have demonstrated that none of the major regimens is convincingly better than CHOP (Fischer et al. 1993; Gordon et al. 1992; Salles et al. 1994). These studies, however, compared multidrug combinations which, in fact, had the same dose intensity as CHOP for the two major agents, adriamycin and cyclophosphamide. Several attempts were made to increase the dosage (Coiffier et al. 1989; Gisselbrecht et al. 1984) and randomized studies are now in progress to evaluate CHOP against a high-dose CHOP regimen such as ACVB. For poor-prognosis lymphoma, however, it is unlikely that a major improvement will be observed. In therapeutic studies the emphasis has now switched to the use of high-dose therapy followed by transplantation of autologous stem cells from peripheral blood or bone marrow (ASCT). Pilot studies of high-dose therapy and ASCT showed that this therapy offers some potential for long-term survival in a limited number of chemosensitive relapsing patients thought to be incurable using conventional therapy (Bosly et al. 1992; Gribben et al. 1989; Philip et al. 1987). However, results from these studies may be misleading, since they are biased notably by the mode of selection of patients; such studies can in no way substitute for prospective comparative trials. Many questions remain unanswered concerning the optimal management of lymphoma and the role of recent technological developments possibly offering new forms of treatment. This review will attempt to summarize the current situation by encompassing all available recent data.

Upfront Autologous Stem Cell Transplantation

The greatest challenge was to identify those patients who ought to be candidates for ASCT because they were unlikely to respond to standard therapy or because their response would be of short duration. The International Non-Hodgkin's Lymphoma Prognostic Factors Project (Shipp et al. 1993) has identified four risk groups based on five pretreatment variables (age, stage, serum LDH, performance status, and number of extranodal disease sites) thereby increasing the likelihood of choosing the optimal treatment for poor-prognosis patients. For patients without adverse factors, the complete remission (CR) rate is 92% and the 5-year survival rate is 83%; these patients represent 22% of the studied population. For those patients with two adverse factors and those with more than two factors, the CR rates are 57% and 46%, and the 5-year survival rates are 46% and 32%, respectively. Such patients represent 46% of the population of patients with aggressive NHL. This subset of patients are the best candidates for studying new strategies.

Several investigators have reported the use of high-dose therapy with autologous BMT as part of the primary therapy of patients with intermediate-grade NHL (Baro et al. 1991; Gulati et al. 1988; Nademanee et al. 1992). Recently, Pettengel et al. (1996) reported a retrospective comparison between standard and intensive treatment strategies for lymphoma patients presenting with two and three prognostic factors according to the International Index. Thirty-four patients received 11 weeks of doxorubicin, cyclophosphamide, vincristine, bleomycin, etoposide, prednisolone, and methotrexate (VAPEC-B), while 33 patients received intensive treatment with 7 weeks of VAPEC-B and three cycles of ifosfamide/cytarabine, followed by high-dose busulfan/cyclophosphamide and then autologous blood progenitor cell support. At 2 years, the rates of event-free survival and overall survival significantly differed between the intensive and standard treatment groups (61% vs 35% and 64% vs 35%, respectively).

These authors concluded that the high-dose therapy approach in high-risk patients was promising but required confirmation using randomized trials. In 1987, the Groupe d'Etude des Lymphomes de l'Adulte (GELA) designed a randomized study to evaluate the potential benefit of a high-dose regimen followed by autologous bone marrow transplantation after CR. Induction treatment was that of the LNH 84 protocol with an open randomization with respect to the anthracycline. After 4 cycles, over a period of 2 months, patients in CR were further randomly assigned to receive either sequential chemotherapy or ASCT. ASCT was performed after a high-dose regimen containing cyclophosphamide, carmustine, and etoposide (CBV). Haioun et al. (1994) reported on 790 patients included in the initial randomization. With a median follow-up duration of 28 months, the 3-year disease-free survival rate was 52% in the sequential chemotherapy arm and 59% in the autologous transplantation arm ($p=0.46$). The 3-year survival rate did not differ between sequential chemotherapy and autotransplantation, i.e., 71% and 69% respectively ($p=0.60$). However, the population enrolled was somewhat heterogeneous. An updated analysis was carried out on 916 eligible patients using the International Index. When applied to patients randomized for consolidation, there was no statistically significant difference between the two consolidation arms, in the low-risk group (0 factor, 110 patients) and in the low-intermediate- and high-risk group (1 factor, 312 patients). On the other hand, for the high-intermediate- and high-risk group (2–3 factors, 236 patients), the 5-year disease-free survival rate was significantly higher in the ASCT arm when compared to chemotherapy (59% vs 39%; $p=0.01$) as well as the 5-year survival rate (65% vs 52%; $p=0.06$). From these different studies, we conclude that dose-intensive consolidation with ASCT should be proposed for patients who achieve CR after induction treatment if they have at least two adverse prognostic factors.

Several randomized studies addressing this question are currently in progress. In one of these, Gianni (1994) developed early intensification with a novel high-dose chemotherapy regimen that takes full advantage of growth factor use. In a phase III trial, a high-dose regimen requiring hematopoietic progenitor cell autotransplantation was randomized with a third-generation chemotherapy regimen (MACOP-B) as the initial treatment for poor-risk non-Hodgkin's lymphoma. In the first interim analysis, 38 patients entered the high-dose arm and 37 patients the MACOP-B arm. After a median follow-up of 43 months, the remission rate (94%) and freedom from progression (88%) were in favor of the intensive arm but overall survival in the latter (73%) was not significantly different from that in the MACOP-B group (62%).

A slow response to conventional chemotherapy is an unfavorable prognostic factor (Armitage et al. 1986). Therefore, another approach would involve selecting patients on the basis of the response after three cycles of chemotherapy. In a randomized phase III study (Verdonck et al. 1995), early application of high-dose chemoradiotherapy and autologous bone marrow transplantation was compared with the continuation of CHOP. Of the 286 patients whose response rate could be evaluated, 38% had fast responses, 47% had slow responses and 15% had no response. Sixty-nine patients with slow responses and without bone marrow involvement were randomized. At 4 years, the rate of event-free survival and overall survival did not significantly differ between the two treatment groups (53% vs 41% and 85% vs 56% respectively, $p>0.10$). The nonrandomized group of fast responders did not differ significantly from those in the randomized study group. Curiously, slow responders randomized to CHOP apparently did better than fast responders, with a 72% event-free survival compared to 54% for the fast responders. This study underlined the difficulty of using early response to treatment as the sole prognostic factors, as well as the need for a large-scale randomized trial in a well-defined group. In aggressive lymphoma with at least two adverse prognostic factors, only 65% of the patients achieved CR with the AVCB regimen. In order to increase the response rate, short, highly intensive therapy (B) with ASCT on day 60 was developed and randomized against the ACVB arm (A) (Gisselbrecht et al. 1996). It consisted of three cycles of chemotherapy and a collection of peripheral blood progenitor cells after the second or third cycle; on day 60, a BEAM regimen was administered, followed by ASCT. Three hundred and two intermediate- or high-grade lymphoma patients were included in the protocol; 35% had three or more adverse factors. CR was observed in 66% for treatment A, and in 67% for treatment B; 23% of the patients did not receive ASCT, mainly due to progression of the disease. The rate of induction failure was similar in both arms. Factors influencing CR were: number of extranodal localizations, bone marrow involvement, and age above 40 years. With a median follow-up of 16 months, event-free survival and overall survival were superior in the conventional chemotherapy arm. From these preliminary data, intensive and short treatment with ASCT did not increase the CR rate compared to ACVB. Early ASCT did not prevent a high, early relapse rate, in contrast to the results obtained when ASCT was performed after remission in this particular group of poor-prognosis patients (Haioun 1995).

Autologous Stem Cell Transplantation in Partial Responders

Achievement of complete remission is the initial goal of induction treatment. The number of cycles needed to achieve CR may vary according to the intensity of chemotherapy, from 6 with the CHOP-like regimen to 4 with ACVB. Patients who achieved only a partial response (PR) to first-line induction therapy represent 5%–15% of de novo aggressive lymphomas. Their outcome is generally poor, and salvage chemotherapy is unable to achieve persistent CR (Bosly et al. 1992). The analysis of the outcome of 93 partial responders under 50 years of age who were treated in the LNH87 study has been reported (Haioun et al. 1995). Histological documentation was available for 57 of the patients (59%). Treatment consisted of salvage chemotherapy followed, in 35 cases, by ASCT. Median time between diagnosis and ASCT was 6 months. For patients treated with ASCT, freedom from progression and survival were, respectively, 58% and 63% – a significant improvement compared to patients treated with conventional treatment only, in whom the 4-year freedom from progression rate was 20% ($p<10^{-4}$) and survival was 46% ($p=0.03$). Martelli et al. (1996) reported a randomized study designed to evaluate, by a second randomization, the effect of DHAP vs ASCT in patients with a partial clinical response after two-thirds of a conventional front-line therapy. A total of 286 patients entered the first randomization trial and 49 the second: 27 in the DHAP arm and 22 in the ASCT arm. In the DHAP group, CR was achieved in 4 (15%) of the patients, while 12 (44%) had a stable PR, and 11 (41%) showed progressive disease. In the ASCT group, 3 (14%) obtained CR, 18 (82%) showed stable PR, and only one progressed. The probability of progression-free survival was 73% for ASCT and 52% for DHAP, and the probability of survival was 73% and 59%, respectively; however, these results did not reach a significant difference. ASCT following aggressive treatment may be more effective than DHAP in reducing the risk of progression in NHL patients with residual lymphoma following first-line therapy. These conflicting results emphasize yet again the need for randomized trials to clarify the situation in aggressive lymphoma. Some subgroups will never need intensive therapy, either because their probability of survival is initially superior to 80%, or because they do not belong in the chemosensitive group. Nevertheless, the selection of patients to be included in a study should be carefully analyzed.

Autologous Stem Cell Transplantation After Relapse

Results of various chemotherapy regimens indicate that over 50% of patients either fail to achieve CR or experience a relapse after a "standard" chemotherapy regimen (Salles et al. 1994). Since fewer than 10% of these patients attain long-term disease-free survival with a salvage chemotherapy regimen, the use of high-dose therapy was investigated in a variety of treatment protocols (Cabanillas et al. 1982; Velasquez et al. 1988). The outcome of salvage chemotherapy is best assessed by examining the three studies that detail the results of IMVP16 (Cabanillas et al. 1982), MIME (Cabanillas et al. 1987) and DHAP (Velasquez et al. 1988). In these salvage studies, projected overall disease-free survival was approximately 15% at 12 months and less than 10% at 2 years for the three trials. Even with the most recent regimen, DHAP, disease-free survival in patients with aggressive lymphoma achieving CR was still only about 25% at 2 years, with no sign of a plateau on the life table plot (Velasquez et al. 1988). Thus, the long-term prognosis for patients given conventional salvage chemotherapy for high- and intermediate-grade lymphomas remains grim. Since the results using various intensive treatments are not convincing, might we expect an improvement with one course of very intensive treatment using hematopoietic stem cell rescue?

High-dose therapy has been most extensively used in patients who have relapsed after conventional therapy. Philip et al. (1987), reporting data on 100 patients from pioneering centers, pointed out three groups of patients with different outcomes following high-dose therapy. Sensitive relapsing patients, after a complete response, had a 3-year disease-free survival of 36%, whereas resistant relapsing or primary refractory patients had disease-free survival of 14% and 0%, respectively. The apparent benefit of intensive therapy with ASCT in sensitive relapse was difficult to confirm because of a bias in the enrollment of patients and the different initial treatment. In order to approach this problem, 244 patients who had undergone unsuccessful therapy or who had relapsed after receiving LNH84 treatment were analyzed to determine the influence of intensive chemotherapy with ASCT upon survival (Bosly et al. 1992). Only 39 of the 180 patients, all under 60 years of age, underwent transplantation, although 115 of them were still responding to salvage chemotherapy. Median overall survival was longer (12.4 vs 6.7 months) for patients treated with bone marrow transplantation, with a 3-year actuarial disease-free survival of 33%. However, only one-third had been considered eligible for intensive treatment (and only 21% of the total population who had had a relapse or unsuccessful treatment). Despite this bias, Cox analysis showed autologous bone marrow transplantation to be an independent significant factor influencing overall survival in patients under the age of 60. It should be noted that the association between different histological subtypes is not uncommon (Robertson et al. 1991), and relapse with a low-grade pattern may be encountered.

Finally, the PARMA randomized trial between high-dose therapy and conventional salvage regimen has now been completed (Philip et al. 1995). A total of 215 patients in the first or second relapse of intermediate- and high-grade NHL were included between July 1987 and July 1994. After two courses of salvage DHAP chemotherapy 109 responding patients were randomized to either four courses of DHAP and radiotherapy (54 patients) or radiotherapy plus high-dose chemotherapy, (BEAC) and ASCT (55 patients). All patients were included in the final analysis: 55 patients were assigned to ASCT and 54 patients to DHAP. The median observation time for randomized patients was 63 months. The response rate after the ASCT procedure was 84%, compared to 44% observed in the DHAP arm. At 5 years, the event-free survival rate was 46% for ASCT vs 12% for DHAP ($p=0.001$). The rate of overall survival was 53% vs 32%, respectively ($p=0.035$). In conclusion, ASCT increases both event-free and overall survival and can be considered a standard treatment for high and intermediate grade NHL in chemosensitive relapse. Prognosis of relapsing patients subjected to ASCT is influenced by several parameters at the time of relapse, including LDH level and the duration of remission (Bosly et al. 1992). For patients relapsing less than 12 months after the diagnosis of lymphoma, the probability of survival at 2 years after ASCT was 19%, whereas for late relapse, survival reached 47%. New approaches for this poor-prognosis group of patients are warranted.

Autologous Stem Cell Transplantation in High-Grade Lymphoma

High-grade NHL are a group of very aggressive malignancies with a rather high incidence of central nervous system (CNS) and bone marrow involvement; they are the most common histologies in pediatric NHL (Murphy et al. 1989). In children, conventional chemotherapy results in long-term disease-free survival in 80% of B cell lymphoma patients and 70% of T cell lymphoma patients (Murphy et al. 1989; Patte et al. 1986). Results in similarly staged adults are unfortunately less successful, for reasons that are unclear.

A review of the literature on adult lymphoblastic lymphoma (LBL) and its treatment by conventional chemotherapy has tended to suggest that patients more than 40 years old with advanced stage IV disease, with either CNS involvement or a significantly raised LDH at presentation, have an especially poor prognosis: less than 20% long-term survival (Coleman et al. 1986; Morel et al. 1992). A retrospective analysis by the European Group for Bone Marrow Transplantation (EBMT) apparently showed different results (Sweetenham et al. 1995). Among the 214 patients reported in the registry, 105 were transplanted in first CR and the 6-year actuarial survival was 63%. Transplantation in second CR resulted in a 31% rate of actuarial survival. These results seem better than those reported for a conventional-dose salvage regimen. In evaluating any chemotherapy series, these poor-prognosis patients must be differentiated from the remainder, who do remarkably well, with over 80% disease-free survival using conventional chemotherapy with standard multiagent-type therapy. Three separate European groups (Milpied et al. 1989; Santini et al. 1991; Verdonck et al. 1992) have shown that the outcome of these poor-risk patients may be improved to around 60% by dose intensification with autologous or allogeneic marrow in a first remission. In the Italian study (Santini et al. 1991), 21 of 40 patients (53%) with lymphoblastic NHL achieved a complete response to sequential chemotherapy and subsequently received high-dose therapy with autologous bone marrow transplantation (BMT). The disease-frese survival was 66% at a median of 58 months. Milpied et al. (1989) treated 25 adults with lymphoblastic NHL in first CR using both autologous ($N=13$) and allogeneic BMT ($N=12$). The disease-free survival at 48 months was 68%, and there were no differences between patients who received autologous and those who received allogeneic BMT. Nine adult patients with poor risk LBL in first remission were treated with non-purged autologous BMB (ABMT) by Verdonck et al. (1992). Six patients are currently in unmaintained first remission with a median follow-up of 53 months. Morel et al. (1992) reported that 5 of 7 patients transplanted in the first CR were alive and event-free 17^{+} to 70^{+} months after BMT. However, overall survival of the 21 transplanted patients in first CR or after relapse was not significantly different from that of the 59 other patients (Morel et al. 1992). Prospective studies are ongoing to overcome the selection bias that such retrospective studies may inadvertently introduce. However, this type of study of transplant vs chemotherapy for such patients has proven difficult to complete due to the rarity of the disease and because these patients may already have had emergency treatment using a variety of protocols before they were referred to the transplant center.

For Burkitt's lymphoma, despite the overwhelming advances in conventional chemotherapy for this disease over the last 15 years, there exist some subgroups of patients with this type of lymphoma who might benefit from ABMT. The group of patients who may benefit from consolidation of first-line therapy are those who achieved a partial response after conventional induction therapy. Data were reported by Philip et al. (1988), who treated 12 children and young adults with high-grade NHL in partial remission with high-dose chemotherapy and autologous BMT. Six of the 12 patients had CNS and/or bone marrow involvement. There was 1 (9%) treatment-related death; 10 of the remaining 11 patients attained CR. At the time these data were presented, disease-free survival was 67% at a mean of 36 months (range 26–94 months).

A retrospective analysis of 117 adult patients reported to the lymphoma registry of the EBMT between June 1984 and November 1994 has been presented (Sweetenham et al. 1994). Seventy of these patients received high-dose therapy and stem cell transplantation in first CR. Data on all patients were reviewed, and prognostic factors were determined by univariate and multivariate analysis. The actuarial overall survival for the entire group was 53% at 3 years. The major factor for predicting outcome after transplantation was disease status: the 3-year actuarial overall survival was 72% for patients undergoing transplantation during the first CR, compared with 37% for patients in chemosensitive relapse and 7% for chemoresistant patients. For patients undergoing transplantation during first CR, disease bulk at the time of ASCT was the only factor predictive of progression-free and overall survival. In most of the retrospective series, these cases clearly represented selection bias, and it must be emphasized that no true prospective randomized study of ABMT in Burkitt's lymphoma has been carried out. Just as with lymphoblastic lymphoma, the number of adult patients and the existence of emergency treatment precludes trials.

Source of Hematopoietic Stem Cells

Patients with bone marrow involvement or who have been compromised by previous cytotoxic therapy and who show myelodysplastic changes may be unsuitable for autologous marrow harvest. For these patients, allogeneic transplantation is advantageous. In eight different series on a total of 154 reported cases of allogeneic transplantation for refractory or relapsed NHL, an event-free probability of 18%–56% was achieved (Lundberg et al. 1991). Moreover, as in leukemia, an allogeneic graft versus lymphoma (GVL) effect was suggested (Jones et al. 1991). Relapse rates in allogeneic transplantation were lower than in autologous transplantation, even after purging treatment. Until now, the decrease in relapses has been assumed to be balanced by the increased mortality due to allogeneic complications (GVH and infections), and no advantage in survival has been observed with allogeneic transplantation. Chopra et al. (1992) reported a case-controlled study of 1060 patients reported to the lymphoma registry of the European Bone Marrow Transplant Group. A total of 938 patients underwent ABMT and 122 patients underwent alloBMT. A case-controlled study was performed by matching 101 alloBMT patients with 101 ABMT patients. Case matching was performed after the selection of the main prognostic factors for progression-free survival by multivariate analysis. Progression-free survival was similar in both types of transplants (49% alloBMT vs 46% ABMT). The overall relapse and progression rate for the alloBMT patients was 23%, compared with 38% in the ABMT patients. This difference was not statistically significant. In the lymphoblastic lymphoma subgroup, alloBMT was associated with a lower relapse rate than ABMT (24% alloBMT v 48% ABMT; $p=0.035$). A significantly lower relapse/progression rate was also observed in patients with chronic graft-vs-host disease (cGVHD) compared with those patients without it (0% cGVHD vs 35% no cGVHD; $p=0.02$). Fourteen of 18 patients who had cGVHD also had lymphoblastic lymphoma. This study suggested that ABMT and alloBMT for non-Hodgkin's lymphoma are comparable, except in lymphoblastic lymphoma, where a graft-vs-lymphoma effect may account for the lower relapse rate in patients who underwent alloBMT.

Peripheral stem cells are now widely used as an alternative source of hematopoietic support (Brice et al. 1996; Vose et al. 1993). The entire process may produce safer results with less morbidity and more efficient use of resources (see Hohaus et al., this volume). A comparison of the outcome of aggressive lymphoma after either ABMT or peripheral blood progenitor cells (PBPC) was made in aggressive lymphoma (Brice et al. 1996; Vose et al. 1993). Retrospective analysis of 105 lymphoma patients without adverse prognostic factors showed that survival was better in patients receiving PBPC (Brice et al. 1996). Another study (Vose et al. 1993) failed to show any advantage in terms of survival for patients treated with intensification and PBPC. Prospective randomized trials may be needed, but will be difficult to achieve because of the dramatic difference in toxicity of PBPC.

Finally, the possible impact of stem cell bone marrow manipulation in vitro deserves further attention. Pharmacological agents and immunological methods with monoclonal antibodies have been used separately or in combination. Because patients with aggressive lymphoma who receive ABMT often relapse after treatment, at their prior sites of disease, it has been claimed that bone marrow purging has no major influence on the outcome. However, recent data suggest that efficient immunological purging may significantly decrease the relapse rate after BMT in bcl-2-positive lymphoid malignancies (Gribben et al. 1991). Sharp et al. (1996) reported that the frequency of relapse after bone marrow or peripheral blood stem cell transplantation is correlated with the presence of lymphoma cells which will grow in appropriate in vitro assays. Although these results must be confirmed in prospective studies, they suggest that the use of purged bone marrow or PBPC may be beneficial. However, these procedures were effective in only half of the cases (Gribben et al. 1991); thus, the relapse rate in autologous transplants may be related in part to the reinfusion of malignant cells.

Conclusion

In the coming years, new tools will appear, enabling us to approach our goal of improving overall survival. It will become easier to test different modalities of high-dose therapy in lymphoma. Most important are the socioeconomic implications of such procedures. Several indications for ASCT have been validated in randomized studies, and should be offered as a standard treatment. The dramatic improvement in terms of toxicity, duration of hospitalization and cost observed after the introduction of peripheral stem cells mobilized by hematopoietic growth factors will obviously facilitate the use of ASCT in standard clinical practice.

References

Armitage JO, Weisenburger DD, Hutchins M et al (1986) Chemotherapy for diffuse large-cell lymphoma – rapidly responding patients have more durable remission. J Clin Oncol 4:160–164

Baro J, Richard C, Calavia J et al (1991) Autologous bone marrow transplantation as consolidation therapy for non-Hodgkin's lymphoma patients with poor prognostic features. Bone Marrow Transplant 8:283–289

Bosly A, Coiffier B, Gisselbrecht C et al (1992) Bone marrow transplantation significantly prolongs survival after relapse in aggressive lymphoma patients treated with the LNH 84 regimen. J Clin Oncol 10:1615–1623

Brice P, Marolleau JP, Pautier P et al (1996) Hematologic recovery and survival of lymphoma patients after autologous stem cell transplantation (ASCT): comparison of bone marrow with peripheral blood progenitor cell (PBSC). Leuk Lymphoma (in press)

Cabanillas F, Hagemeister FB, Bodey GP et al (1982) IMVP 16: an effective regimen for patients with lymphoma who have relapsed after initial combination chemotherapy. Blood 60:693–697

Cabanillas F, Hagemeister FB, McLaughlin P et al (1987) Results of MIME salvage regimen for recurrent or refractory lymphoma. J Clin Oncol 3:407–412

Chopra R, Goldstone AH, Pearce R et al (1992) Autologous versus allogenic bone marrow transplantation for non-Hodgkin's lymphoma: a case-controlled analysis of the European Bone Marrow Transplant Group registry data. J Clin Oncol 10:1690–1695
Coiffier B, Gisselbrecht C, Herbrecht R et al (1989) LNH84 regimen: a multicenter study of intensive chemotherapy in 737 patients with aggressive malignant lymphoma. J Clin Oncol 7:1018–1026
Coleman CN, Picozzi VJ, Cox RS et al (1986) Treatment of lymphoblastic lymphoma in adults. J Clin Oncol 4:399–404
Fisher RI, Gaynor E, Dahlberg S et al (1993) Comparison of a standard regimen (CHOP) with three intensive chemotherapy regiments for advanced non-Hodgkin's lymphoma. N Engl J Med 328:1002–1006
Gianni AM (1994) 5-Year update of the Milan Cancer Institute randomized trial of high-dose sequential (HDS) vs MACOP-B therapy for diffuse large-cell lymphomas. Proc Am Soc Clin Oncol 13:373
Gisselbrecht C, Lepage E, Fermand JP et al (1984) Intensive induction treatment in non-Hodgkin lymphomas with various grades of malignancy. In: Sotto, Vroussos, Vincent (eds) Cancer research workshop, Grenoble. Karger, Basel, pp 195–199
Gisselbrecht C, Lepage E, Morel P et al (1996) Short and intensified treatment with autologous stem cell transplantation (ASCT) versus ACVB regimen in poor prognosis aggressive lymphoma (Abstr). Br J Haematol 93:561
Gordon LI, Harrington DP, Andersen J et al (1992) Comparison of a second generation combination chemotherapeutic regimen (m-BACOD) with a standard regimen (CHOP) for advanced diffuse non-Hodgkin's lymphoma. N Engl J Med 327:1342–1349
Gribben JG, Goldstone AH, Linch DC et al (1989) Effectiveness of high-dose combination chemotherapy and autologous bone marrow transplantation for patients with non-Hodgkin's lymphoma who are still responsive to conventional-dose therapy. J Clin Oncol 7:1621–1629
Gribben JG, Freedman AS, Neuberg D et al (1991) Immunologic purging of marrow assessed by PCR before autologous bone marrow transplantation for B-cell lymphoma. N Engl J Med 325:1525–1533
Gulati SC, Shank B, Black P et al (1988) Autologous bone marrow transplantation for patients with poor prognosis lymphoma. J Clin Oncol 6:1303–1313
Haioun C (1995) Autologous bone marrow transplantation (ABMT) versus sequential chemotherapy for aggressive non-Hodgkin's lymphoma (NHL) in first complete remission (CR): a study of 542 patients (LNH87-2 protocol) (Abstr). Blood 86:1816
Haioun C, Lepage E, Gisselbrecht C et al (1994) Comparison of autologous bone marrow transplantation with sequential chemotherapy for intermediate and high grade non-Hodgkin's lymphoma in first complete remission. A study of 464 patients. J Clin Oncol 12:2543–2551
Haioun C, Lepage E, Gisselbrecht C et al (1995) Autologous transplantation versus conventional salvage therapy in aggressive non-Hodgkin's lymphoma (NHL) partially responding to first line chemotherapy. Study of 96 patients enrolled in the LNH87-2 protocol (Abstr). Blood 86:833
Jones RJ, Ambinder RF, Piantadosi S et al (1991) Evidence of a graft versus lymphoma effect associated with allogenic bone marrow transplantation. Blood 77:649–653
Lundberg JH, Hansen RM, Chitambar CR et al (1991) Allogenic bone marrow transplantation for relapsed and refractory lymphoma using genotypically HLA identical and alternative donors. J Clin Oncol 9:1848–1859
Martelli M, Vignetti M, Zinzani PL et al (1996) High-dose chemotherapy followed by autologous bone marrow transplantation versus dexamethasone, cisplatin, and cytarabine in aggressive non-Hodgkin's lymphoma with partial response to front-line chemotherapy: a prospective randomized Italian multicenter study. J Clin Oncol 14:534–542
Milpied N, Ifrah N, Kuentz M et al (1989) Bone marrow transplantation for adult poor prognosis lymphoblastic lymphoma in first complete remission. Br J Haematol 73:82–87
Morel P, Lepage E, Brice P et al (1992) Prognosis and treatment of lymphoblastic lymphoma in adults: a report on 80 patients. J Clin Oncol 10:1078–1085

Murphy SB, Fairclough DL, Hutchinson RE et al (1989) Non-Hodgkin's lymphoma of childhood: an analysis of the histology, staging and response to treatment of 338 cases at a single institution. J Clin Oncol 7:186–193

Nademanee A, Schmidt G, O'Donnell MR et al (1992) High dose chemoradiotherapy followed by autologous bone marrow transplantation as consolidation therapy during first complete remission in adult patients with poor-risk aggressive lymphoma: a pilot study. Blood 80:1130–1134

Patte C, Philip T, Rodary C et al (1986) Improved survival rate in children with stage III and IV B-cell non-Hodgkin's lymphoma and leukemia using multi-agent chemotherapy: results of a study of 114 children from the French Pediatric Oncology Society. J Clin Oncol 4:1219–1226

Pettengel R, Radford JA, Morgenstern GR et al (1996) Survival benefit from progenitor-cell transplantation in poor-prognosis non-Hodgkin's lymphoma. J Clin Oncol 14:586–592

Philip T, Armitage JO, Spitzer G et al (1987) High dose therapy and autologous bone marrow transplantation after failure of conventional chemotherapy in adults with intermediate-grade or high grade non-Hodgkin's lymphoma. N Engl J Med 316:1493–1498

Philip T, Hartman O, Biron P et al (1988) High dose therapy and autologous bone marrow transplantation in partial remission after first-line induction therapy for diffuse non-Hodgkin's lymphoma. J Clin Oncol 6:1118–1124

Philip I, Guglielmi C, Hagenbeek A et al (1995) A prospective randomized study comparing autologous bone marrow transplantation (ABMT) and salvage chemotherapy (DHAP) in sensitive relapse on non-Hodgkin's lymphoma (NHL): final analysis of the PARMA study. N Engl J Med 333:1540–1545

Robertson LE, Redman JR, Bulter JJ et al (1991) Discordant bone marrow involvement in diffuse large-cell lymphoma: a distinct clinical-pathologic entity associated with a continuous risk of relapse. J Clin Oncol 9:236–242

Salles G, Shipp MA, Coiffier B (1994) Chemotherapy of non-Hodgkin's aggressive lymphomas. Semin Hematol 31:46–69

Santini G, Congui AM, Coser P et al (1991) Autologous bone marrow transplantation for adult advanced stage adult lymphoblastic lymphoma in first CR: a study of the NHLGSG. Leukemia 5 Suppl 1:42–45

Sharp JG, Kessinger A, Mann S et al (1996) Outcome of high-dose therapy and autologous transplantation in non-Hodgkin's lymphoma based on the presence of tumor in the marrow or infused hematopoietic harvest. J Clin Oncol 14:214–219

Shipp MA, Harrington DP, Anderson JR et al (1993) Development of a predictive model for aggressive lymphoma: the international Non-Hodgkin's Lymphoma Prognostic Factors Project. N Engl J Med 329:987–994

Sweetenham JW, Liberti G, Pearce R et al (1994) High-dose therapy and autologous bone marrow transplantation for adult patients with lymphoblastic lymphoma: results of the European Group for Bone Marrow Transplantation. J Clin Oncol 12:1358–1365

Sweetenham JW, Pearce R, Taghipour G et al (1995) Adult Burkitt's and Burkitt-line non-Hodgkin's lymphoma (NHL) favourable outcome for patients undergoing high dose therapy and autologous stem cell transplantation (ASCT) in first remission or chemosensitive relapse: results from the EBMT (Abstr). Blood 86:832

Velasquez WS, Cabanillas F, Salvadore P et al (1988) Effective salvage therapy for lymphoma with cisplatin in combination with high dose Ara C and dexamethasone (DHAP). Blood 71:117

Verdonck LF, Dekker AW, Gijsbert C et al (1992) Autologous bone marrow transplantation for adult poor-risk lymphoblastic lymphoma in first remission. J Clin Oncol 10:644–646

Verdonck LF, Van Putten WLJ, Hagenbeek A et al (1995) Comparison of CHOP chemotherapy with autologous bone marrow transplantation for slowly responding patients with aggressive non-Hodgkin's lymphoma. N Engl J Med 332:1045–1092

Vose MJ, Anderson JR, Kessinger A et al (1993) High dose chemotherapy and autologous hematopoietic stem cell transplantation for aggressive non-Hodgkin's lymphoma. J Clin Oncol 11:1846–1851

Peripheral Blood Progenitor Cell Transplantation in Multiple Myeloma Following High-Dose Melphalan-Based Therapy

H. Goldschmidt[1], U. Hegenbart[1], M. Wallmeier[1], S. Hohaus[1], R. Engenhart[2], M. Wannenmacher[2], and R. Haas[1]

[1] Department of Internal Medicine V, University of Heidelberg, Hospitalstraße 3, 69115 Heidelberg, Germany
[2] Department of Radiology, University of Heidelberg, Im Neuenheimer Feld 400, 69120 Heidelberg, Germany

Abstract

The objective of our study was to evaluate the efficacy and toxicity of a high-dose melphalan-based therapy with or without total body irradiation (TBI) followed by peripheral blood progenitor cell (PBPC) transplantation in patients with multiple myeloma. Between June 1992 and June 1996, 104 patients (71 male, 33 female) with a median age of 51 years (range 30–65 years) underwent transplantation at our center. PBPC were mobilized using high-dose chemotherapy followed by treatment with G-CSF. Fifty patients were treated with TBI+melphalan 140 mg/m^2 while 54 patients received melphalan 200 mg/m^2. Following PBPC autografting, the median time to attainment of platelets $\geq 20\times10^9$/l and neutrophils $\geq 0.5\times10^9$/l was 11 and 14 days, with no difference between the treatment groups. In the TBI group significantly longer periods of total parenteral nutrition were required due to the occurrence of severe mucositis. Two patients from the TBI group died of transplantation-related complications. Following high-dose treatment, remission state improved in 43 out of 102 patients. No statistically significant advantage in reaching complete or partial remission was observed with TBI+high-dose melphalan compared to the treatment with high-dose melphalan alone. The optimal high-dose treatment, with particular reference to the inclusion or omission of TBI, should be prospectively investigated.

Introduction

Multiple myeloma is a B-cell disorder with a median survival of 3 years when conventional chemotherapy is used (Alexanian and Dimopoulos 1994). Most randomized trials have failed to show an improvement in survival by using combination chemotherapy instead of melphalan with or without prednisone (Samson 1996; Gregory et al. 1992). A promising treatment approach for multiple myeloma is based on reports of high complete remission rates after the administration of dose-escalated alkylating agents, which was piloted by T.J. McElwain in the early 1980s using high-dose melphalan (McEl-

Recent Results in Cancer Research, Vol. 144

wain and Powles 1983). Hematopoietic progenitor cell transplantation allows a further increase in the dose of cytotoxic drugs and the addition of total body irradiation (TBI). The final results of the randomized IFM 90 study showed significantly longer event-free survival and overall survival with high-dose melphalan and TBI followed by autologous bone marrow transplantation in comparison with conventionally treated patients (Attal et al. 1996). We present our single-center experience of 104 patients with multiple myeloma who were included in a high-dose treatment program with peripheral blood progenitor cell (PBPC) transplantation.

Patients and Methods

From June 1992 to June 1996, 104 patients with multiple myeloma were enrolled in this study. Inclusion criteria were (1) multiple myeloma defined as stage III according to the Durie-Salmon classification (Durie and Salmon 1975) or progressive stage II disease, (2) age below 65 years, (3) creatinine clearance above 60 ml/min, (4) normal electrocardiogram (ECG), stress ECG and echocardiogram, (5) no cardiac arrhythmias equal or greater than Lown IV B in the Holter ECG, and (6) normal liver function (serum bilirubin <2.0 g/dl alanine transaminase and aspartate transaminase <3×normal value) and no disease progression during conventional polychemotherapy. Seventy-one patients were male and 33 female; the median age was 51 years (range 30–65 years). Patient characteristics are shown in Table 1. At our center, patients were treated with VAD (vincristine, Adriamycine, dexamethasone) or VBMCP (M 2 protocol; vincristine, BCNU, melphalan, cyclophosphamide, prednisone) until the paraprotein level reached a plateau or complete remission by European Bone Marrow Transplant Group (EBMTG) criteria (Attal 1993) was achieved. Patients referred from other hospitals had been pretreated with melphalan/prednisone ($n=43$) or other chemotherapy regimens ($n=4$). To improve their remission status, 37 of these 47 patients received at least three cycles of VAD. The median number of previous chemotherapy cycles was seven (range 3–28), and 42 out of the 104 patients had a history of previous irradiation. Most patients had advanced disease (79 patients with stage III). Three patients with symptoms of the disease were in stage I and were included on their own request. Complete (CR) and partial remission (PR) were defined according to the EBMTG criteria, according, to which, for PR, a 50% reduction of the M-component in serum or 75% reduction of urine paraprotein is required, while CR requires normal serum protein electrophoresis, proteinuria below 0.25 g/l and less than 5% plasma cells in the bone marrow. A negative immunofixation was not necessary for CR classification.

PBPC Mobilization

To mobilize PBPCs and to reduce the tumor load before high-dose melphalan-containing therapy, 91 patients received high-dose cyclophosphamide

Table 1. Patient characteristics in the two treatment groups ($n=104$)

	TBI+140 mg/m² melphalan ($n=50$)	200 mg/m² melphalan ($n=54$)	p value
Age (years) (median; range)	50; 30–60	53; 40–65	0.0062
Male/female ratio	32/18	39/15	0.3681
Paraprotein type			
No. of patiens with type G/A/BJ/D	28/13/7/1	30/8/12/2	0.5234
No. of asecretory patients	1	2	
No. of patients with stage I/II/III, disease	3/11/36	0/10/44	0.1573
No. of patients with stage B disease	7 patients	12 patients	0.2783
No. of previous therapy cycles (median; range)	7; 3–28	8; 3–25	0.8600
No. of patients with previous radiation	18	26	0.2103
No. of patients with β_2-microglobulin ≥6 g/l[a]	4	3	0.9160
No. of patients with β_2-microglobuline ≥2.5 g/l[a]	13	15	0.9864
No. of patients with Hypercalcemia[a]	8	10	0.9364

[a] At diagnosis

(HD-cy, 15 patients 4 g/m², 76 patients 7 g/m² cyclophospamide or, for patients with preexisting heart disease or amyloidosis, ifosfamide/mitoxantrone (13 patients). Twenty-four hours after chemotherapy, filgrastim (R-metHuG-CSF, 300 μg/day, Amgen-Roche, Munich, Germany) administration was commenced to increase the number of circulating hematopoietic progenitor cells during leukocyte recovery. Administration was continued until PBPC harvesting was completed. Measurements of circulating CD 34+ cells were begun when the white blood cell count reached a level of greater than 1.0×10^9/l. PBPC collection was initiated when a distinct population of CD 34+ cells (CD 34+>10 cells/μl) could be detected in the peripheral blood (see Hohaus et al., this volume).

Collection of PBPCs and Cryopreservation Procedure

Harvesting was performed with a Fenwal CS 300 (Baxter Deutschland, Munich, Germany) or with a Cobe Spectra (Cobe, Lakewood, Colorado, USA). For each leukapheresis, 10–20 l blood was processed at a flow rate of 50–150 ml/min using large-bore central venous catheters as previously described (Murce et al. 1997). The apheresis product of a 50-ml cell suspension was mixed with the same volume of minimal essential medium containing 20% dimethyl-sulfoxide (DMSO; Merck, Darmstadt, Germany). The final 100-ml cell suspension was transferred into freezing bags (Delmed, New Brunswick, New Jersey, USA) and frozen to –100 °C using a computer-controlled cryopreservation device (Cryoson BV-6; Cryoson Deutschland, Germany). The frozen cells were transferred into liquid-phase nitrogen and stored at –196 °C. The PBPC mobilization and collection was considered successful if a minimum of 2.0×10^6 CD 34+ cells/kg body weight were harvested.

Clonogenic Assay for Hematopoietic Progenitor Cells

The concentration of hematopoietic progenitor cells in each individual leukapheresis product and in the peripheral blood was assessed using a semisolid clonogenic culture assay (Terry Fox Laboratories, Vancouver, Canada) as previously described (Hohaus et al. 1993).

Immunofluorescence Staining and Flow Cytometry

For immunofluorescence analysis, 20 µl whole blood or 1×10^6 mononuclear cells were incubated for 30 min at 4 °C with the fluorescein isothiocyanate (FITC)-conjugated monoclonal antibody (moAb HPCA-2 (anti-CD 34; Becton Dickinson, Heidelberg, Germany) and analyzed using a Becton Dickinson FACScan as previously described (Hohaus et al. 1993).

Pretransplantation Conditioning Regimen and Intensive Care After Transplantation

In 50 patients, the pretransplantation conditioning therapy consisted of TBI (14.4 Gy, hyperfractionated over 4 days) and 140 mg/m^2 melphalan or, in 54 patients, of 200 mg/m^2 melphalan alone, because of previous spinal radiotherapy, reduced pulmonary diffusion capacity, or refusal to undergo TBI. Following high-dose conditioning therapy, PBPCs were reinfused without additional bone marrow or growth factor support. Patients received prophylactic bowel decontamination, and antibiotic combination therapy was administered for fever above 38.5 °C, while amphotericin-B was added if there was documented fungal infection or persistent fever. A platelet count greater than 20×10^9/l was maintained by ABO-matched platelet transfusions, and packed red blood cells were given when the hemoglobin level was less than 8 g/dl.

Statistical Analysis

The clinical and laboratory data from the patients were evaluated according to standard statistical methods using a commercially available computer program (Statistica for Windows, Stat Soft, Tulsa, Oklahoma, USA).

Results

PBPC Collection and Autografting with G-CSF-Mobilized PBPCs

PBPCs were harvested in a median of three leukaphereses (range 1–10) resulting in 3.3×10^6 CD34+ cells/kg body weight (median; range 1.5×10^6–58.3×10^6 CD34+ cells/kg body weight). Autografts contained beween 1.5×10^6 and 29.0×10^6 CD34+ cells/kg body weight (median 3.3) and between 4.0 and 181.4×10^4 CFU-C/kg body weight (median 15.45). Only one patient received an autograft of less than 2.0×10^6 CD34+ cells/kg body weight. A neutrophil count of 0.5×10^9/l was reached after a median of 14 days, with a range from 8 to 31 days. Platelets recovered rapidly, reaching an increasing unsubstituted count of more than 20×10^9/l between 4 and 157 days (median 11) after transplantation. Neutrophil and platelet recovery were not different following TBI+melphalan compared to the treatment with high dose melphalan alone. The hematological reconstitution is shown as cumulative frequency in Fig. 1, while the nonhematological toxicity is shown in Table 2. More days with fever and antibiotic as well as antimycotic treatment were observed after TBI. In the TBI group, significantly longer periods of parenteral nutrition were also necessary due to severe mucositis. The increased number of platelet and erythrocyte transfusion is caused by the shorter survival of blood cells dur-

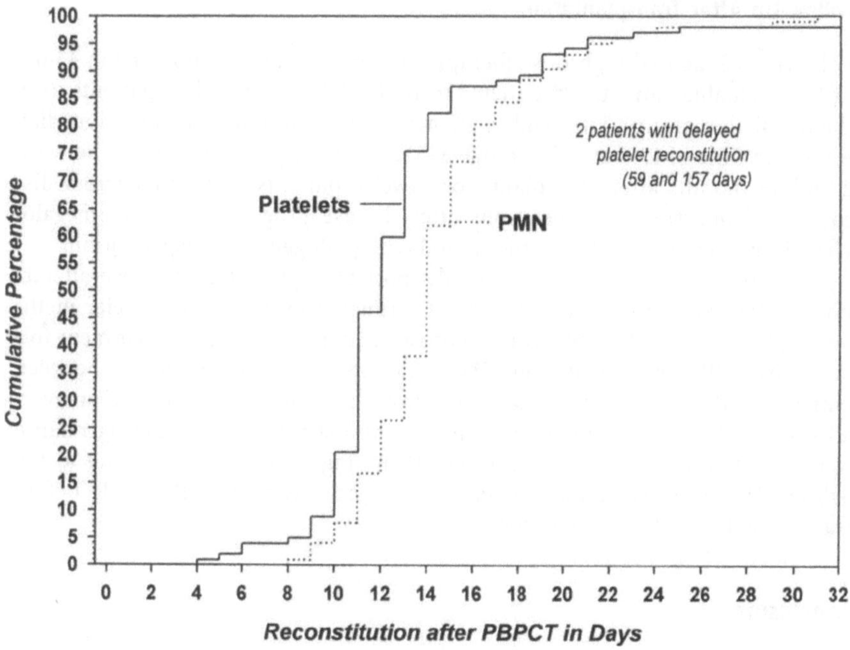

Fig. 1. Reconstitution of neutrophils and platelets after peripheral blood progenitor cell transplantation (PBPCT) in 104 patients with multiple myeloma

Table 2. Toxicity following high-dose therapy with peripheral blood progenitor cell transplantation (medians and ranges)

	TBI+140 mg/m^2 melphalan (n=50)	200 mg/m^2 melphalan (n=54)	p value
Days with fever >38.5°C	4 (1–11)	1 (0–9)	<0.0001
Days of antibiotic treatment	12 (6–27)	6 (0–41)	<0.0001
Days of antimycotic treatment	0 (0–15)	0 (0–0)	0.0003
Days of total parenteral nutrition	11 (2–22)	0 (0–26)	<0.0001
No. of platelet transfusions	4 (1–16)	1 (0–50)	<0.0001
No. of erythrocyte transfusions	2.5 (0–10)	2 (0–8)	0.0495
Days in hospital	18 (12–58)	17 (12–39)	0.2085

ing fever. Because hematological reconstitution was the same in both treatment groups, there was no difference in hospitalization time.

Two transplantation-related deaths were observed in the TBI group (one patients with sepsis and multiorgan failure at day 23 and a second patient with cardiac failure 13 days after transplantation).

Follow-Up After Transplantation

Following sequential high-dose therapy, the remission state improved in 43 out of 102 evaluable patients (27 patients from the TBI group and 15 patients from the melphalan group). Fifty-eight patients are alive in remission after a median follow-up time of 17.0 months (range 3–51), while 41 patients relapsed between 2 and 43 months after transplantation. Twelve patients died of recurrent disease, 4 of infectious complications after disease progression, 1 cytomegalovirus infection, and 1 of pneumonia following allogeneic transplantation.

Event-free survival is 50% 22 months post-transplantation and overall survival is 68% after 36 months (Fig. 2) as estimated by the Kaplan-Meier method. A plateau event-free survival is not reached after high-dose treatment followed by PBPC transplantation. There was no significant difference between patients in the TBI or melphalan-only group in regard to event-free or overall survival (Fig. 3). In our patient group, the main factors predicting relapse were elevated β2-microglobulin, stage III or stage B disease according to the Salmon-Durie classification, hypercalcemia, not reaching CR or PR before transplantation, and IgA subtype.

Conclusion

In patients with multiple myeloma, high-dose therapies have been shown to improve remission rates compared to conventional treatment. The final anal-

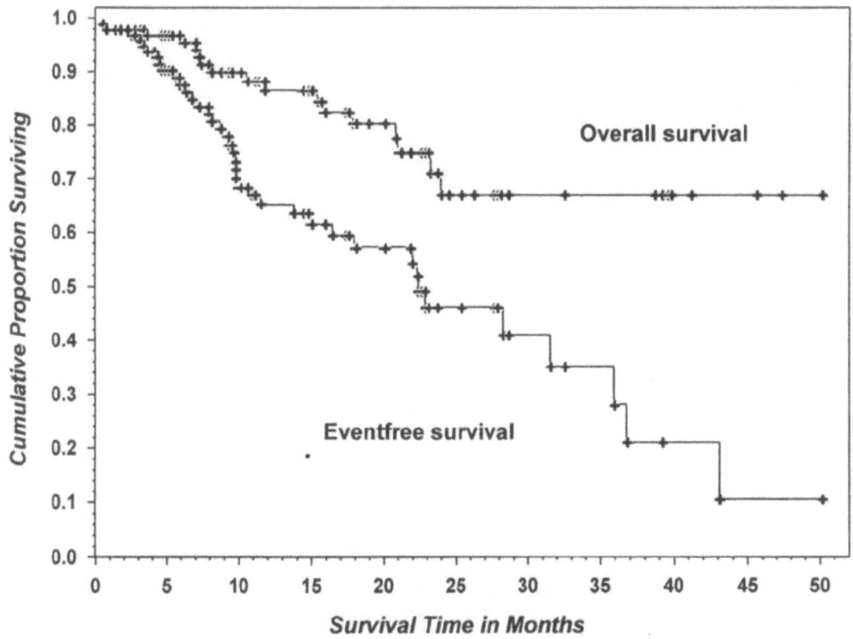

Fig. 2. Overall and event-free survival after PBPCT in 104 patients with multiple myeloma

ysis of the French multicenter trial IFM 90 showed a significantly longer event-free and overall survival following high-dose treatment (Attal et al. 1996). Similar results were presented in 1995 by Barlogie et al. at the ASH meeting. The data from the Royal Marsden group (Cunningham et al. 1994) show that high-dose melphalan is the most active agent in the treatment of multiple myeloma. With particular reference to the inclusion or omission of TBI in the high-dose approach, data are only available in regard to small patient groups. In a retrospective analysis of 85 patients, the remission state in chemosensitive patients was better with TBI+high-dose melphalan than with high-dose melphalan alone (Jagannath and Barlogie 1992). In treatment-refractory patients, the toxicity of TBI-containing treatment is up to 20% (Vesole et al. 1994). No randomized study comparing TBI plus chemotherapy with high-dose melphalan has yet been carried out (Mohrbacher and Anderson 1995).

Our results in 104 patients show no advantage of the TBI-containing high-dose therapy over the treatment with high-dose melphalan but without TBI in achieving PR or CR. Treatment-related toxicity, on the other hand, was significantly increased in the TBI group, in which the two deaths due to toxicity occurred. Prospective randomized studies are required to address the question of the optimal high-dose regimen prior to transplantation of autologous PBPCs in patients with multiple myeloma.

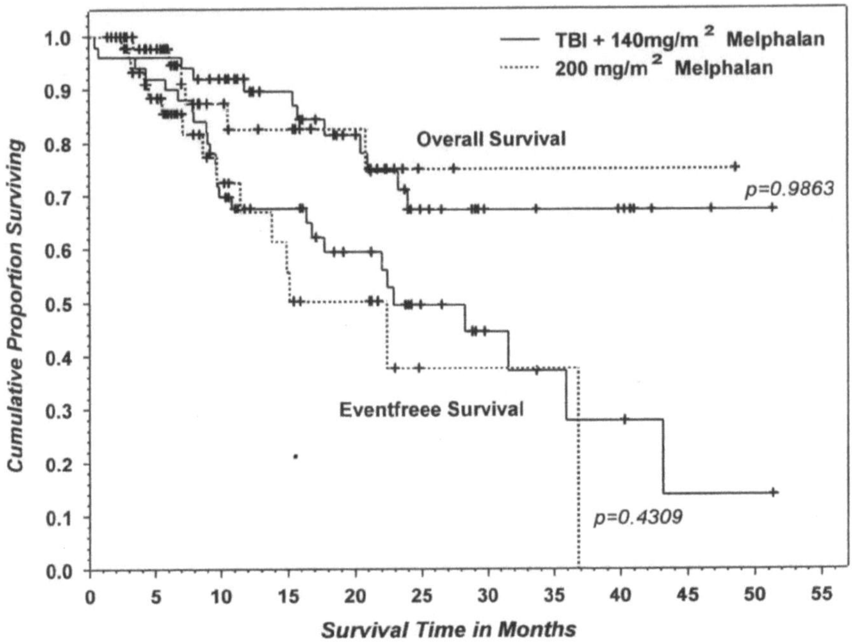

Fig. 3. Overall and event-free survival after PBPCT in 104 patients with multiple myeloma, by treatment group

Acknowledgements. The authors thank the nursing staff of the Bone Marrow Transplantation Unit and of the ward "Station Vierordt" for their outstanding care of these patients, and Margit Pförsich, Kirsten Flentje, Evi Holdermann, Magdalena Volk for their excellent technical assistance. We are indebted to Prof. Meuer (Institute for Immunology and Serology, University of Heidelberg) and his colleagues for providing the packed erythrocyte and ABO-matched platelet transfusion. We are gratefully to Dr. David Maclachlan, MRCGP, for reading the manuscript.

References

Alexanian R, Dimopoulos M (1994) The treatment of multiple myeloma. N Engl J Med 330:484–489

Attal M (1993) A randomized study testing the effect of bone marrow/peripheral blood stem cell transplantation or conventional chemotherapy, with or without alpha interferon for aggressive myeloma. EORTC Leukemia Cooperative Group, EBMT Myeloma Study Group, French Myeloma Study Groups (GEM-POF), study protocol

Attal M, Harousseau JL, Stoppa et al (1996) High dose therapy in multiple myeloma: final analysis of a prospective randomized study of the "Intergroup Francais du Myeloma" (IFM 90). N Engl J Med 335:91–97

Barlogie B, Crowley J, Jagannath S et al (1995) Superior outcome after early autotransplantation (AT) with "Total Therapy" (TT) compared to standard SWOG treatment (ST) for multiple myeloma (MM) (Abstr). Blood 86:207 a

Cunningham D, Paz-Ares L, Milan S et al (1994) High-dose melphalan and autologous bone marrow transplantation as consolidation in previously untreated myeloma. J Clin Oncol 12:759–763

Durie B, Salmon S (1975) A clinical staging system for multiple myeloma. Cancer 36:842–852

Gregory WM, Richards MA, Malpas JS (1992) Combination therapy versus melphalan and prednisolone in the treatment of multiple myeloma: an overview of published trials. J Clin Oncol 10:334–342

Hohaus S, Goldschmidt H, Ehrhardt R et al (1993) Successful autografting following myeloablative conditioning therapy with blood stem cells mobilized by chemotherapy plus rhG-CSF. Exp Hematol 21:508–514

Jagannath S, Barlogie B (1992) Autologous bone marrow transplantation for multiple myeloma. Hematol Oncol Clin North Am 6:451–462

McElwain TJ, Powles RL (1983) High dose intravenous melphalan for plasma cell leukemia and myeloma. Lancet 2:822–824

Mohrbacher A, Anderson KC (1995) Bone marrow transplantation in multiple myeloma. In: Malpas JS, Bergsagel DE, Kyle RA (eds) Myeloma. Biology and management. Oxford University Press, Oxford, pp 322–352

Murea S, Goldschmidt H, Hahn U et al (1997) Successful collection and transplantation of peripheral blood stem cells in cancer patients using large-volume leukapheresis. J Clin Apheresis 11:185–194

Samson D (1996) Principles of chemotherapy and radiotherapy. In: Gahrton M, Durie BGM (eds) Multiple myeloma. Arnold, London, pp 108–129

Vesole DH, Barlogie B, Jagannath S et al (1994) High-dose therapy for refractory multiple myeloma: improved prognosis with better supportive care and double transplants. Blood 84:950–956

Molecular Monitoring of Residual Disease in Chronic Myelogenous Leukemia Patients After Therapy

A. Hochhaus, A. Reiter, H. Skladny, A. Reichert, S. Saußele, and R. Hehlmann

Third Medical Clinic, University of Heidelberg, Wiesbadener Straße 7–11, 68305, Mannheim, Germany

Abstract

The degree of tumor load reduction after therapy, which is determined by the degrees of cytoreduction and cytogenetic response, is an important prognostic factor for patients with chronic myelogenous leukemia (CML). Conventional metaphase analysis is considered to be the "gold standard" for evaluating cytogenetic response. The frequency of cytogenetic analysis can be reduced considerably if patients are monitored by molecular methods, such as quantitative Southern blot, fluorescence in situ hybridization (FISH), quantitative western blot, or competitive reverse transcriptase polymerase chain reaction (RT-PCR). Molecular methods can be performed on peripheral blood specimens and are therefore less invasive than cytogenetic analyses of bone marrow metaphases. Furthermore these techniques are applicable to Ph-negative/BCR-AbL-positive cases. Results obtained by Southern blotting, western blotting, and FISH are readily quantifiable but their sensitivity is not generally superior to that of cytogenetic methods. RT-PCR is by far the most sensitive method. Quantitative RT-PCR analysis is the method of choice for monitoring patients after bone marrow transplantation (BMT). Using competitive PCR in patients after BMT, reappearance and/or rising levels of BCR-ABL transcripts can be detected prior to relapse. All complete cytogenetic responders to interferon-α are positive for BCR-ABL transcripts. The level of residual disease spans a range over found orders of magnitude. In both interferon-α-treated patients and patients after BMT a good correlation between BCR-ABL transcript numbers per microgram of RNA and cytogenetic results has been found. Variables in the competitive PCR assay may be controlled for by quantification of transcripts of the normal ABL gene as an internal standard. We suggest a stepwise strategy for diagnosis and follow-up of CML patients employing molecular methods.

Introduction

Chronic myelogenous leukemia (CML) is characterized in about 90% of cases by the presence of a shortened chromosome 22, the Philadelphia (Ph) chromosome. The molecular background is the reciprocal translocation of genetic

Recent Results in Cancer Research, Vol. 144

material between the BCR gene on chromosome 22 and the ABL gene on chromosome 9. The resulting chimeric BCR-ABL fusion gene is transcribed to a specific BCR-ABL mRNA, which in most patients encodes a 210-kDa chimeric protein with increased tyrosine kinase activity. The crucial role of BCR-ABL in several pathways which lead to uncontrolled proliferation has been shown in vitro and in vivo by transfection experiments in mice (reviewed in Gordon and Goldman 1996).

The efficacy of interferon-*α* (IFN-*α*) in CML, as monotherapy or in combination with chemotherapeutic drugs, has been demonstrated in several randomized trials (Allan et al. 1995; Italian Cooperative Study Group on Chronic Myeloid Leukemia 1994; Hehlmann et al. 1994; Ohnishi et al. 1995). IFN-*α* induces hematologic responses in 60%–80% of cases and cytogenetic responses, i.e., suppression of the Ph-positive clone, in up to 55% of patients. It has been suggested that the amount of residual tumor burden after therapy correlates inversely with prolongation of survival (Kantarjian et al. 1995; Mahon et al., this volume).

Currently, allogeneic bone marrow transplantation is the only therapeutic approach with the intention to cure CML patients. This method, however, is available for only 30% of patients, due to age restrictions and restrictions in the availability of HLA-matched donors (Mughal and Goldman 1995).

Conventional methods for monitoring the tumor burden CML patients on therapy are white blood cell number and cytogenetic analysis of bone marrow metaphases. The latter method, however, is limited by the mitotic cell requirement. Insufficient metaphases are obtained from many patients on IFN-*α* therapy. Furthermore, cytogenetic analysis is not applicable to patients with Ph-negative/BCR-ABL-positive disease. We sought to establish molecular methods at the DNA and RNA levels to monitor CML patients on IFN-*α* therapy. The aims of our study were (i) to standardize the detection of the BCR-ABL fusion gene, (ii) to quantify residual disease in patients after therapy, and (iii) to correlate the cytogenetic results with molecular data.

Methods for Detecting and Quantifying BCR-ABL

The conventional method for monitoring patient response to therapy is the cytogenetic analysis of bone marrow metaphases. The generally accepted classification of the cytogenetic response follows the Houston definition (Kantarjian et al. 1995):

- Complete response (0% Ph-positive metaphases)
- Partial response (1%–34% Ph-positive metaphases)
- Minor response (35%–94% Ph-positive metaphases)
- No response (≥95% Ph-positive metaphases)

Molecular methods by which to detect the BCR-ABL fusion gene are:

- Southern blot at the DNA level
- Fluorescence in situ hybridization (FISH) at the chromosomal/DNA level
- Western blot at the protein level
- Reverse transcriptase polymerase chain reaction (RT-PCR) at the RNA level

Southern Blot Analysis

Using a set of appropriate enzymes and probes, a BCR rearrangement located in the major breakpoint cluster region (M-bcr) is detectable in about 98% of Ph-positive cases (de Klein et al. 1986). For routine use, *Bgl* II and *Xba* I are appropriate restriction enzymes, informative in almost all cases. In rare instances, however, Southern blot analysis is negative due to breakpoints outside M-bcr or mutations of the affected BCR allele (Bartram et al. 1987; Saglio et al. 1990; Pane et al. 1996; Hochhaus et al. 1996a; Melo 1996).

Using densitometry of the autoradiograph signals, Southern blot facilitates quantification of the proportion of cells, out of all cells investigated, that carry a BCR rearrangement. The "BCR ratio" has been established to express this proportion: [BCR ratio = (2×rearranged signals)/(rearranged+germline signals)]. Quantitative Southern blot allows detection and quantification of as little as 1% leukemic cells (Verschraegen et al. 1995; Reiter et al. 1995; Grossman et al. 1991; Westbrook 1996).

DNA from 235 blood and marrow samples from CML patients was analyzed by quantitative Southern blot. The results were compared with the proportion of Ph-positive metaphases found in contemporaneous bone marrow specimens analyzed by conventional cytogenetic analysis. The rank correlation between the two methods was $r = 0.82$ ($p < 0.001$). BCR ratios were significantly different between cytogenetically defined minor, partial, and complete response groups ($p < 0.0001$). Empirically derived cut-off points in the BCR ratio were introduced in order to define molecular response groups: a BCR ratio of 0% was defined as complete response, and ratios of 1%–24%, 25%–50%, and >50% were defined as showing partial, minor, and no molecular response, respectively. Using these groupings, a major cytogenetic response could be predicted or excluded in more than 90% of cases (Reiter et al. 1995, 1997).

Fluorescence In Situ Hybridization

Dual color-FISH using probes for BCR and ABL genes allows specific detection of the BCR-ABL gene fusion in interphase and/or metaphase nuclei. A limitation of this method is the background of about 2% false-positive cells (Bentz et al. 1994). However, FISH is applicable for quantification of residual disease in partial, minor, and nonresponders to IFN-α (Cox Froncillo et al. 1996).

Western Blot

The BCR-ABL western blot assay allows quantification of the BCR-ABL protein both in bone marrow and in peripheral blood. As little as 1% of Ph-positive cells can be detected. The western blot assay can distinguish two kinds of BCR-ABL proteins, p210 and p185. The Houston group found a linear correlation between BCR-ABL/ABL protein ratios and contemporaneous conventional cytogenetic analysis in 392 sample pairs ($r=0.97$, $p<0.001$) (Guo et al. 1994, 1996).

Multiplex RT-PCR

A further approach is the detection of specific mRNA transcripts by RT-PCR. For diagnostic samples, the use of multiplex PCR has been suggested to detect simultaneously several kinds of BCR-ABL and BCR transcripts as internal controls in one reaction (Cross et al. 1994a). This method allows the detection of typical BCR-ABL transcripts, such as b2a2 or b3a2, and atypical fusions, e.g., transcripts lacking ABL exon a2 (b2a3 and b3a3) or transcripts resulting from BCR breakpoints outside M-bcr, such as e1a2 or e6a2 (Hochhaus et al. 1996a).

Minimal Residual Disease

The methods described have a maximum sensitivity of 1%, i.e., a patient with negative cytogenetic analysis, Southern blot, western blot, or multiplex RT-PCR results may harbor up to 10^{10} residual leukemic cells (Fig. 1).

The term "minimal residual disease" refers to the presence of detectable malignant cells in patients who are in conventional (cytogenetics, Southern blot, western blot) remission. The aim of minimal residual disease analysis is to distinguish patients who have differing levels of residual leukemic cells and who may therefore benefit from either reduced or intensified treatment regimens. By nested RT-PCR, CML cells remaining after treatment can be

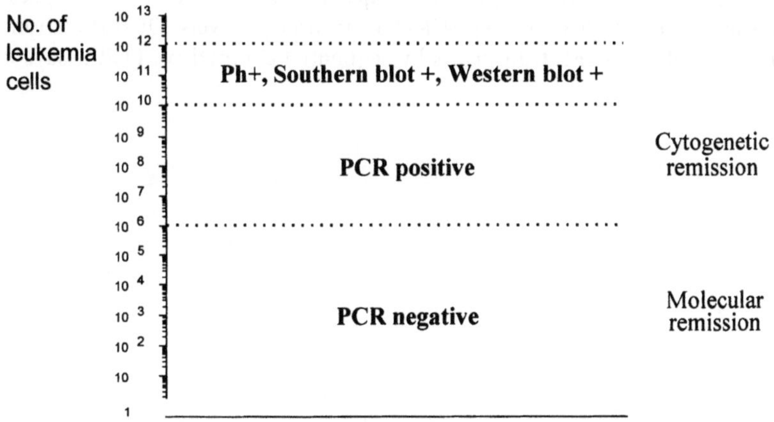

Fig. 1. Levels of remission. Patients in conventional (cytogenetic, Southern blot, western blot) remission may harbor up to 10^{10} residual leukemic cells. Nested RT-PCR is able to detect minimal residual disease up to a level of 10^6 cells in the body

specifically detected with a sensitivity of up to 1 in 10^6 cells. PCR is performed after reverse transcription of RNA using nested primers corresponding to appropriate BCR and ABL exons. This qualitative method has been used for the detection of minimal residual disease after bone marrow transplantation (BMT). A summary of 700 results from 15 centers shows that

- The majority of patients are PCR-positive in the first 6 months after BMT.
- The graft-versus-leukemia effect causes PCR negativity in two-thirds of patients; persistent PCR-negativity more than 1 year after BMT is a marker of a good prognosis.
- PCR-positive patients more than 6 months after BMT are at great risk of relapse.
- Qualitative PCR cannot predict relapse in the individual patient (Cross et al. 1993, 1994b; Potter et al. 1993).

Quantitative PCR

On the basis of the above findings, we employ a competitive PCR method to quantify residual BCR-ABL transcripts. Nested PCR is performed using serial dilutions of a BCR-ABL competitor construct added to the same volume of patients cDNA (Fig. 2). The equivalence point at which the competitor and sample band would be of equal intensity is determined by densitometry (Cross et al. 1993; Hochhaus et al. 1996b). In order to standardize results for both quality and quantity of blood, RNA, and cDNA, quantification of transcripts of the normal ABL gene is used; the standardized result is expressed as the ratio BCR-ABL/ABL in percent. Quantification of the transcript level of normal genes is of particular importance if different RNA qualities are expected, especially if samples from multicenter trials are mailed to a reference laboratory.

Following up patients *after allogeneic BMT*, out of 69 patients with low or falling BCR-ABL transcripts 3% relapsed, compared to 79% relapses in 29 patients with high or rising BCR-ABL transcript levels. Quantification of the number of BCR-ABL transcripts by sequential competitive PCR assays can de-

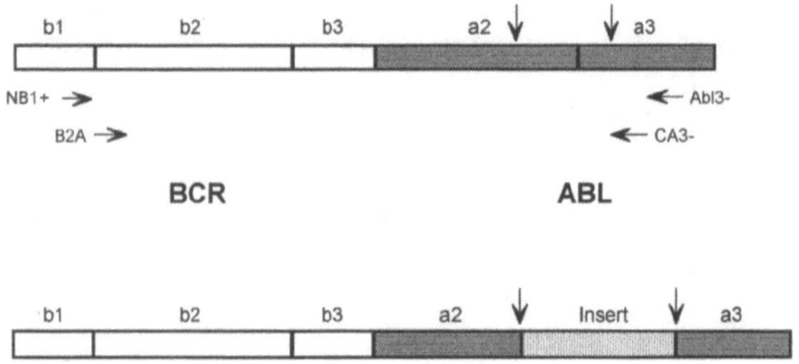

Fig. 2. b3a2 BCR-ABL transcript and p210-BCR-ABL competitor construct. Nested PCR is performed using serial dilutions of the competitor added to the same volume of patient's cDNA

tect increasing numbers of leukemia-specific transcripts in the individual patient with a proliferating leukemia cell population (Cross et al. 1994b; Lin et al. 1996).

Quantitative PCR is the method of choice for determining the best time-point for therapeutic interventions in cases of relapse after BMT. Early *administration of donor lymphocytes* prior to hematologic relapse improves the response rate (van Rhee et al. 1994).

Out of 96 Ph-positive patients who had received IFN-α *therapy*, all were positive for BCR-ABL transcripts. The result is expressed as the ratio of the number of BCR-ABL and ABL transcripts in percent. The residual disease in complete responders spans a range over four orders of magnitude. The median ratios in complete, partial, minor, and nonresponders differ significantly ($p<0.0001$). There is no difference between the results of nonresponders on IFN-α therapy and those of patients at diagnosis (Fig. 3) (Hochhaus et al. 1995, 1996b).

During follow-up, 6 out of 29 complete cytogenetic responders relapsed; three relapsed with reappearance of the Ph-positive clone in chronic phase, while three developed a blast crisis without preceding cytogenetic relapse. During complete remission the patients who subsequently relapsed showed relatively high BCR-ABL/ABL ratios. Residual disease resides in myeloid colony-forming cells which may have the potential to repopulate the bone marrow and contribute to relapse. Therefore, it is unlikely that CML can be cured by IFN-α therapy.

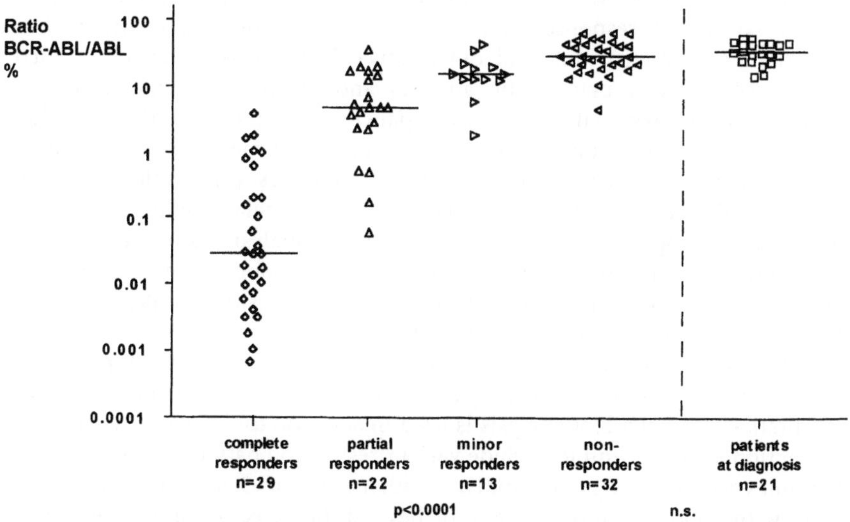

Fig. 3. BCR-ABL/ABL ratios of 96 Ph-positive CML patients on IFN-α therapy. Results are significantly different between the cytogenetic response groups ($p<0.0001$). All complete cytogenetic responders on IFN-α therapy were RT-PCR-positive. Their residual BCR-ABL/ABL ratios span a range over four order of magnitude

Cytogenetic response to IFN-α (complete, partial, minor/none) was compared to molecular response by introducing cut-off points for the BCR-ABL/ABL ratio. Using optimum cut-off points of 2% and 14%, i.e., comparing a ratio of up to 2% to complete cytogenetic responders, between 2% and 14% to partial responders, and greater than 14% to minor and nonresponders, the concordance between the two methods was 82% and the χ^2 test was highly significant ($p<0.001$).

Strategy for Molecular Response Monitoring

The degree of response to therapy, i.e., the residual tumor burden, is an important prognostic indicator. The question of how best to monitor response to treatment is still controversial. Whilst cytogenetic detection of the proportion of marrow metaphases lacking a Ph chromosome remains the "gold standard" by which all other tests are judged, little attention is generally paid to the pitfalls of this method of analysis. In particular, the statistical significance of sampling small numbers of metaphases (Hook 1977) and the effects of culture conditions are not generally appreciated. Molecular methods may offer some advantages for monitoring patients with CML. Quantitative Southern blot, quantitative FISH, quantitative western blot, and competitive RT-PCR can be performed on peripheral blood specimens and are therefore less invasive than conventional cytogenetic analysis of bone marrow. Furthermore, these techniques are applicable to Ph-negative/BCR-ABL-positive cases.

We have shown that BCR-ABL transcript numbers/μg RNA and BCR-ABL/ABL ratios correlate with the cytogenetic response. Using optimum cut-off points, equivalent response groups can be defined for cytogenetic analysis, quantitative Southern blot, and quantitative PCR. However, an exact correspondence between cytogenetic analysis and molecular methods was not found. Possible explanations for discrepancies are, first, that the reproducibility of cytogenetic data depends on the number of metaphases analyzed: in some IFN-α-treated patients the number of metaphases available for analysis is restricted. Second, cytogenetic analysis and molecular methods investigate different cell populations. Whereas cytogenetic analysis examines only cultured myeloid cells in mitosis, competitive PCR, quantitative Southern blot, and quantitative western blot measure amounts of residual leukemia-specific RNA, DNA, or protein of all cells tested.

Currently we are pursuing the following strategy. To detect the type of BCR-ABL fusion in newly diagnosed patients we are performing multiplex PCR. Qualitative Southern blot analysis is used in addition to determine informative restriction enzymes and to exclude variant restriction patterns. In IFN-α-based therapies we are using quantitative Southern blot at 3-monthly intervals. In cases with good responses close to or beyond the detection limit, competitive PCR is performed in addition. Quantitative PCR is the method of choice to monitor complete cytogenetic responders and patients who have undergone allogeneic BMT, or donor lymphocyte transfusions. Patients who have re-

Table 1. Strategy for molecular response monitoring using quantitative Southern blot (Q-SB) and quantitative polymerase chain reaction (Q-PCR)

	Q-SB	Q-PCR
Follow-up on IFN-α therapy	+++	++
Complete cytogenetic responders after IFN-α	+	+++
Follow-up after allogenous BMT	–	+++
Monitoring after donor lymphocyte transfusion	+	++
Monitoring after intensive chemotherapy, autologous BMT or stem cell transplantation	+	++

+++ Method of choice; ++ appropriate method; + appropriate method for a certain period of time; – inappropriate method

ceived autologous stem cells or bone marrow can be monitored by quantitative PCR and/or quantitative PCR (Table 1).

In combination with quantification of normal genes, competitive PCR is applicable even if the sample quality is variable. We employ quantification of ABL transcript numbers to check for possible variation in the quantity and quality of blood, RNA, and cDNA samples. The quantification of internal standards is of particular importance in multicenter studies due to the degradation of RNA during mailing, but it is also useful to check for variables in routine competitive PCR analysis.

For patients who show significant changes in the BCR-ABL/ABL transcript ratio or the BCR ratio, cytogenetic analysis should be done in addition. Only cytogenetic analysis can detect additional chromosomal aberrations which could indicate impending acceleration prior to clinical manifestation. The combination of cytogenetic analysis and quantitative molecular methods may significantly improve the ability to assess response to therapy in patients with CML.

Acknowledgments. The competitive PCR method was established by Dr. N.C.P. Cross, London, UK. We are grateful to Prof. J.M. Goldman, London, UK, for continuous generous support. The study was supported by the Dr. Mildred Scheel Stiftung and the Forschungsfonds, Fakultät für Klinische Medizin Mannheim, Universität Heidelberg. The M-bcr probes for Southern blot analysis were provided by Professor Bartram, Heidelberg, Germany. We thank the clinicians and cytogeneticists participating in the German CML trials and in the UK Medical Research Council CML trials for sending samples and providing clinical and cytogenetic data.

References

Allan NC, Richards SM, Shepherd PC (1995) UK Medical Research Council randomised, multicentre trial of interferon-alpha n1 for chronic myeloid leukaemia: improved survival irrespective of cytogenetic response. The UK Medical Research Council's Working Parties for Therapeutic Trials in Adult Leukaemia. Lancet 345:1392–1397

Bartram CR, Bross Bach U, Schmidt H, Waller HD (1987) Philadelphia-positive chronic myelogenous leukemia with breakpoint 5′ of the breakpoint cluster region but within the bcr gene. Blut 55:505–511

Bentz M, Cabot G, Moos M, Speicher MR, Ganser A, Lichter P, Dohner H (1994) Detection of chimeric BCR-ABL genes on bone marrow samples and blood smears in chronic myeloid and acute lymphoblastic leukemia by in situ hybridization. Blood 83:1922–1928

Cox Froncillo MC, Maffei L, Cantonetti M, Del Poeta G, Lentini R, Bruno A, Masi M, Tribalto M, Amadori S (1996) FISH analysis for CML monitoring? Ann Hematol 73:113–119

Cross NCP, Feng L, Chase A, Bungey J, Hughes TP, Goldman JM (1993) Competitive polymerase chain reaction to estimate the number of BCR-ABL transcripts in chronic myeloid leukemia patients after bone marrow transplantation. Blood 82:1929–1936

Cross NCP, Melo JV, Goldman JM (1994a) An optimized multiplex polymerase chain reaction (PCR) for detection of BCR-ABL fusion mRNAs in haematological disorders. Leukemia 8:186–189

Cross NCP, Feng L, Zhang JG, Goldman JM (1994b) Competitive PCR to monitor residual disease after bone marrow transplantation for chronic myeloid leukaemia. In: Borden EC, Goldman JM, Grignani F (eds) Molecular diagnosis and monitoring of leukaemia and lymphoma. Ares-Serono Symposia Publications, pp 119–126

De Klein A, Hagemeijer A, Bartram CR, Houwen R, Hoefsloot L, Carbonell F, Chan L, Barnett M, Greaves M, Kleihauer E et al (1986) bcr rearrangement and translocation of the c-abl oncogene in Philadelphia positive acute lymphoblastic leukemia. Blood 68:1369–1375

Gordon MY, Goldman JM (1996) Cellular and molecular mechanisms in chronic myeloid leukaemia: biology and treatment. Br J Haematol 95:10–20

Grossman A, Silver RT, Szatroswki TP, Gutfriend A, Verma RS, Benn PA, (1991) Densitometric analysis of Southern blot autoradiographs and its application to monitoring patients with chronic myeloid leukemia. Leukemia 5:540–547

Guo JQ, Lian JY, Xian YM, Lee MS, Deisseroth AB, Stass SA, Champlin RE, Talpaz M, Wang JY, Arlinghaus RB (1994) BCR-ABL protein expression in peripheral blood cells of chronic myelogenous leukemia patients undergoing therapy. Blood 83:3629–3637

Guo JQ, Lian J, Glassman A, Talpaz M, Kantarjian H, Deisseroth AB, Arlinghaus RB (1996) Comparison of *bcr-abl* protein expression and Philadelphia chromosome analyses in chronic myelogenous leukemia patients. Am J Clin Pathol 106:442–448

Hehlmann R, Heimpel H, Hasford J, Kolb HJ, Pralle H, Hossfeld DK, Queisser W, Loffler H, Hochhaus A, Heinze B et al (1994) Randomized comparison of interferon-alpha with busulfan and hydroxyurea in chronic myelogenous leukemia. Blood 84:4064–4077

Hochhaus A, Lin F, Reiter A, Skladny H, van Rhee F, Shepherd PCA, Allan NC, Hehlmann R, Goldman JM, Cross NCP (1995) Variable numbers of BCR-ABL transcripts persist in CML patients who achieve complete cytogenetic remission with interferon-α. Br J Haematol 91:126–131

Hochhaus A, Reiter A, Skladny H, Melo JV, Sick C, Berger U, Guo JQ, Arlinghaus RB, Hehlmann R, Goldman JM, Cross NCP (1996a) A novel BCR-ABL fusion gene (e6a2) in a patient with Philadelphia chromosome negative chronic myelogenous leukemia. Blood 88:2236–2240

Hochhaus A, Lin F, Reiter A, Skladny H, Mason PJ, van Rhee F, Shepherd PCA, Allan NC, Hehlmann R, Goldman JM, Cross NCP (1996b) Quantification of residual disease in chronic myelogenous leukemia patients on interferon-α therapy by competitive polymerase chain reaction. Blood 87:1549–1555

Hook EB (1977) Exclusion of chromosomal mosaicism: tables of 90%, 95%, and 99% confidence limits and comments on use. Am J Hum Genet 29:94–97

Italian Cooperative Study Group on Chronic Myeloid Leukemia (1994) Interferon alfa-2a as compared with conventional chemotherapy for the treatment of chronic myeloid leukemia. N Engl J Med 330:820–825

Kantarjian HM, Smith TL, O'Brien S, Beran M, Pierce S, Talpaz M, and the Leukemia Service (1995) Prolonged survival in chronic myelogenous leukemia after cytogenetic response to interferon-α therapy. Ann Intern Med 122:254–261

Lin F, van Rhee F, Goldman JM, Cross NCP (1996) Kinetics of increasing BCR-ABL transcript numbers in chronic myeloid leukemia patients who relapse after bone marrow transplantation. Blood 87:4473–4478

Melo JV (1996) The diversity of BCR-ABL fusion proteins and their relationship to leukemia phenotype. Blood 88:2375–2384

Mughal TI, Goldman JM (1995) Chronic myeloid leukaemia: a therapeutic challenge. Ann Oncol 6:637–644

Ohnishi K, Ohno R, Tomonaga M, Kamada N, Onozawa K, Kuramoto A, Dohy H, Mizoguchi H, Miyawaki S, Tsubaki K et al (1995) A randomized trial comparing interferon-alpha with busulfan for newly diagnosed chronic myelogenous leukemia in chronic phase. Blood 86:906–916

Pane F, Frigeri F, Sindona M, Luciano L, Ferrara F, Cimino R, Meloni G, Saglio G, Salvatore F, Rotoli B (1996) Neutrophilic-chronic myelogenous leukemia (CML-N): a distinct disease with a specific marker (BCR-ABL with c3a2 junction). Blood 88:2410–2414

Potter MN, Cross NCP, van Dongen JJ, Saglio G, Oakhill A, Bartram CR, Goldman JM (1993) Molecular evidence of minimal residual disease after treatment for leukaemia and lymphoma: an updated meeting report and review. Leukemia 7:1302–1314

Reiter A, Skladny H, Hochhaus A, Schultheis B, Bartram CR, Heimpel H, Hehlmann R (1995) Comparison between cytogenetics and quantitative Southern blot analysis for monitoring interferon α treatment CML-patients (Abstr). Blood 86 Suppl 1:527a

Reiter A, Skladny H, Hochhaus A, Seifarth W, Bartram CR, Heimpel H, Cross NCP, Hehlmann R (1997) Quantitative Southern blot for monitoring CML patients on therapy. Br J Haematol 97:86–93

Saglio G, Guerrasio A, Rosso C, Zaccaria A, Tassinari A, Serra A, Rege Cambrin G, Mazza U, Gavosto F (1990) New type of Bcr/Abl junction in Philadelphia chromosome-positive chronic myelogenous leukemia. Blood 76:1819–1824

Van Rhee F, Lin F, Cullis JO, Spencer A, Cross NCP, Chase A, Garicochea B, Bungey J, Barrett J, Goldman JM (1994) Relapse of chronic myeloid leukemia after allogeneic bone marrow transplant: the case for giving donor leukocyte transfusions before the onset of hematologic relapse. Blood 83:3377–3383

Verschraegen CF, Talpaz M, Hirsch Ginsberg CF, Pherwani R, Rios MB, Stass SA, Kantarjian HM (1995) Quantification of the breakpoint cluster region rearrangement for clinical monitoring in Philadelphia chromosme-positive chronic myeloid leukemia. Blood 85:2705–2710

Westbrook CA (1996) Debate round table: Monitoring of residual disease in chronic myelogenous leukemia: methodological approaches and clinical aspects. Comments. Leukemia 10:905–906

Delineation of Genomic Regions in Chromosome Band 7q22 Commonly Deleted in Myeloid Leukemias

K. Fischer[1], J. Brown[1], S.W. Scherer[2], P. Schramm[1], J. Stewart[3], G. Fugazza[4], U. Pascheberg[5], W. Peter[5], L.-C. Tsui[2], P. Lichter[6], and H. Döhner[1]

[1] Department of Internal Medicine V, University of Heidelberg, Hospitalstraße 3, 69115 Heidelberg, Germany
[2] Department of Genetics, The Hospital for Sick Children, Toronto, Ontario, Canada
[3] Duncan Guthrie Institute of Medical Genetics, Glasgow, Scotland
[4] Department of Internal Medicine, University of Genoa, Genoa, Italy
[5] Institute of Laboratory Medicine, Dortmund, Germany
[6] Department "Organisation of Complex Genomes", German Cancer Research Center, Im Neuenheimer Fel 28 D, Heidelberg, Germany

Introduction

Malignant hematological disorders are characterized by recurring chromosome abnormalities (Mitelman et al. 1995). These chromosome aberrations offer insights into the pathogenesis of these tumors. To date, the major emphasis has been put on the molecular analysis of the recurring translocations, which are though to result in the activation of an oncogene in a dominant fashion, either by deregulating the expression of an oncogene or via the formation of a novel fusion gene (Rabbits 1994).

However, the loss of genetic material in human tumors has also received considerable interest. Such a loss may result from chromosome monosomy or chromosome deletion as well as other genetic mechanisms. In myeloid disorders, such as myelodysplastic syndrome (MDS) and acute myeloid leukemia (AML), these chromosome deletions cluster in a few regions of the genome: the long arm of chromosome 5 (5q), 7q, 9q, 11q, 13q, 20q, and the short arm of chromosome 12 (12p) (Johannsson et al. 1993; Mitelman et al. 1995). The recurring loss of chromosome material suggests that the inactivation of tumor suppressor genes is involved in the pathogenesis of these malignant hematological diseases. Moreover, this observation provides a starting point for the positional cloning of a number of tumor suppressor genes.

Monosomy 7 (-7) or deletion of its long arm (7q-) are among the most frequent aberrations leading to loss of chromosome material in myeloid leukemias (Fourth International Workshop on Chromosomes in Leukemia 1982). These aberrations are associated with both MDS and AML, in particular with therapy-related MDS/AML (t-MDS/t-AML) following therapy with alkylating agents, or secondary MDS/AML after occupational or environmental exposure to chemical mutagens such as benzene, petroleum, and other organic solvents (Mitelman et al. 1978; Le Beau et al. 1986). -7/7q- are observed in approximately 10% of the patients with MDS/AML arising de novo and are

Recent Results in Cancer Research, Vol. 144

much more frequent in the patients with secondary MDS/AML. In a recent series of 246 consecutive cases with t-MDS/t-AML published by Le Beau et al. (1996), 127 (52%) tumors exhibited abnormalities of chromosome 7. Furthermore, -7/7q- occur in MDS and AML which develop in patients with constitutional disorders (e.g., Fanconi's anemia, Kostmann's syndrome, neurofibromatosis type 1, familial monosomy 7) (Luna-Fineman et al. 1995). Clinically, myeloid leukemias exhibiting -7/7q- are associated with high susceptibility to infections, poor response to chemotherapy, and short survival times (Bloomfield and de la Chapelle 1987).

These data are consistent with the hypothesis that inactivation of a tumor suppressor gene located on 7q is a common event that contributes to the pathogenesis of malignant myeloid disorders.

Delineation of 7q Aberrations Using Chromosome Banding Analysis

The delineation of a commonly deleted segment on 7q has been more difficult than that of deletions of other chromosomes, because loss of a whole chromosome 7 represents the most common abnormality and fewer myeloid tumors are available for analysis which exhibit an interstitial or a terminal deletion of 7q. Based on chromosome banding analysis, there appear to be two critical regions on the long arm of chromosome 7, one region in band 7q22 and a second, less frequently involved region in bands 7q32–q33.

To delineate these critical regions on 7q, Le Beau et al. (1996) analyzed the breakpoints of 7q deletions in 81 myeloid tumors (t-MDS/t-AML, $n=26$; de novo MDS or AML, $n=55$). The majority had the proximal deletion breakpoints in bands 7q11–q22 (65 of 81, 80%). The distal breakpoints in these cases varied from band 7q22 to band 1q36 (7q36=35; 7q22=10; 7q34=10; others=10). The tumors which had the proximal breakpoints in band 7q22 and the tumors which had the distal breakpoints in 7q22 allowed these investigators to delineate the commonly deleted region to band 7q22. Furthermore, nine tumors were identified which exhibited balanced translocations involving band 7q22, providing further evidence that a commonly deleted segment is located in this chromosome band. Sixteen of the 81 tumors had more distal deletions. The proximal deletion breakpoints were located to bands 7q31 ($n=5$) or 7q32 ($n=11$) and the distal breakpoints to bands 7q33 to 7q36. Thus, the commonly deleted region of these distal deletions was delineated to bands 7q32–q33.

Rodrigues et al. (1996) analyzed 54 patients with MDS/AML and deletions of the long arm of chromosome 7 using chromosome banding analysis. Concordant with the study of Le Beau et al. (1996), loss of band 7q22 was the most common event. Forty of the 54 (74%) tumors had a 7q22 deletion; the remaining 14 tumors had more distal deletions. The commonly deleted region of the distal deletions was delineated to bands 7q31–q33.

In our own study (Fischer et al. 1997), we analyzed the breakpoints of deletions and translocations involving or encompassing band 7q22 in 21 patients with myeloid disorders [chronic myeloid leukemia (CML) = 2; MDS = 4; AML = 15] using G-banding analysis. Concordant with previous studies, we localized the commonly deleted segment of these deletions to chromosome band 7q22. Furthermore, we identified one MDS and one AML case which exhibited a balanced translocation involving band 7q22.

Molecular Delineation of 7q Aberrations

At present, data on the molecular characterization of the genomic regions affected by these deletions are scarce. No tumor suppressor gene of pathogenetic significance has yet been identified. To delineate the critical region in band 7q22 at the molecular level, different methods have been applied, including restriction fragment length polymorphism (RFLP) analysis, quantitative Southern blot analysis, and fluorescence in situ hybridization (FISH).

Kere et al. (1989a) studied four patients with myeloid disorders exhibiting partial 7q deletions. Using RFLP and quantitative Southern blot analysis, they localized the proximal breakpoints of all four cases between the genes encoding erythropoietin (*EPO*) and plasminogen activator inhibitor 1 (*PLANH1*), which map approximately 3 centimorgans (cM) apart at 7q21.3–q22. To define the distal deletion breakpoints, Kere et al. (1989b) used DNA probes recognizing the *MET* oncogene at 7q31, the *TCRB* locus at 7q34–q35, and a few probes identifying genomic sequences of unknown function at 7q31-qter. All deletions were interstitial with a variability of the distal breakpoints. In another RFLP study, Lewes et al. (1996) analyzed five patients with myeloid disorders and 7q deletions. They used 11 different DNA probes which were distributed over the long arm of chromosome 7. All five deletions were interstitial, with a great variability of the proximal and distal breakpoints. However, in all these studies the resolution of the deletion map was limited, since the applied probes were scattered along a large genomic region.

To delineate the commonly deleted segment in band 7q22 at the molecular level more precisely, several groups have recently applied FISH using contiguously mapped DNA probes from this chromosome region (Johnson et al. 1996; Le Beau et al. 1996; Fischer et al. 1997). We previously reported on a series of 21 patients with various myeloid leukemias (Fischer et al. 1997). We now have extended this series to 28 tumors (CML, $n=2$; de novo MDS, $n=5$; de novo AML, $n=18$, t-AML, $n=3$) which on chromosome banding analysis exhibited deletions ($n=26$) or reciprocal translocations ($n=2$) of band 7q22. As probes for FISH we used 22 yeast artificial chromosome (YAC) clones which span chromosome bands 7q21.3–q23, including representative clones from a panel of YACs recognizing a contiguous genomic DNA fragment of 5–6 Mb in band 7q22 (Scherer et al. 1992, 1994; Kunz et al. 1994; Tsui et al. 1995). In the 26 cases with deletions, we identified two distinct commonly deleted regions: one region within band 7q22 was defined by the two CML cases and is approximately 2–3 Mb in size; the second region encompassed

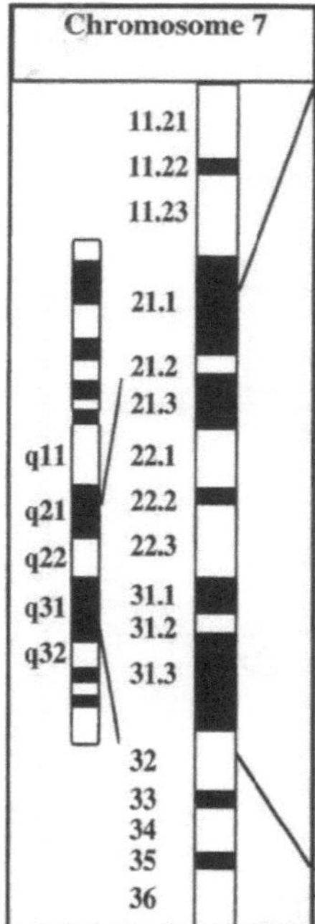

Band		D-marker	CML 1	CML 2	MDS 3	MDS 4	MDS 5	MDS 6	MDS 7	AML 8	AML 9	AML 10	AML 11	AML 12	AML 13	AML 14	AML 15	AML 16	AML 17	AML 18	AML 19	AML 20	AML 21	AML 22	AML 23	AML 24	AML 25	t-AML 26	t-AML 27	t-AML 28
7q21.1		*D7S581*	del	di	di	di	di	del		di	del	di	di	di	di	del	del	di	di	di	del			di		di		del	del	
7q21.1-q21.2		*D7S166*	del							di	del			di	di	del	del	del						di		di		del		
7q21.1-q21.3		*D7S269*	del	di	di	di	di			di	del	di	di	di	di	del	del	del	di	di	del	di		di	del	del	7q	del	del	
7q21.1-q21.3		*D7S183*										di										di	di				3q			
7q21.3		*D7S15*	del	di	del	di	del			di	del	del	di	di	di	del	del	del	di	di		del		del				del		
7q21.3-q22.1		*D7S82*					del			di		del	del	del	di		del		di	di	del		del	del		del		del	del	
7q22		*D7S651*	del	di	del	di	del			di	del		del	del		del	del	del	di	di										
7q22	Contig*	*D7S647*	del	di	del	di	del	del		di	del	del	del	del	di	del	del	del	di	di	del							del	del	di
7q22	Contig*	*D7S2832*		del						di					di															di
7q22	Contig*	*D7S477*	del	del	del	di	del			del	del	del	del	del	del	del	del	del	del	di				del				del		del
7q22	Contig*	*D7S515*	del	del	del	del	del			del	del	del	del	del	del	del	del	del	del	di	del							del	del	del
7q22	Contig*	*D7S2448*	del	di																di										
7q22	Contig*	*942E8.18*	del	di		del	del				del								del	del						del		del		del
7q22	Contig*	*D7S658*	di	di	del	del				del	del	del	del	del	del	del	del	del	del	del					del			del	del	del
7q22	Contig*	*D7S818*	di	di		del				del	del	del				del			del	del								del		
7q22	Contig*	*D7S2509*	di	di	del	del				del	del	del	del	del	del	del	del	del	del	del	del							del	del	
7q22.3-q31.1	Contig*	*D7S2494*	di	di	del	del	del	del	3	del	del	del	del	del	del	del	del	del	del	del	del				del			del	del	
7q22.3-q31.1		*D7S496*	di	di	del	del	del	del		del	del	del	del	del	del	del	del	del	del	del	del	del	del	del	del			del	del	del
7q22.3-q31.1		*D7S13*	di	di	del	del	del			del	del	del	del	del	del	del	del	del	del	del	del			del				del	del	
7q31.2-q31.3		*D7S567*	di	di	del	del	del			del	del	del	del	del	del	del	del	del	del	del	del	del				del		del	del	del
7q31.3-q32.1		*D7S480*			del	del	del			del	del	del	del	del	del	del	del	del	del	del	del			di				del	del	
7q32.1		*D7S514*			del	del	del	del		del	del	del	di	del	del	del	del	del	del	del	del	del	del	di	del	del		del	del	del
7q36		*D7S68*	di	di	di	del	di			di	di	di	di	del	del	del	di	del	di	del	del	di	del					del	del	di

Fig. 1. Mapping of deletions and translocations involving chromosome band 7q22 in 28 myeloid leukemias by FISH. The *light gray* boxes indicate the extent of the deletion in the individual tumor. The *dark gray* boxes indicate the two commonly deleted segments in CML and MDS/AML, respectively. *Empty boxes:* not done. *CML*, Chronic myeloid leukemia; *MDS*, myelodysplastic syndrome; *AML*, acute myeloid leukemia; *t-AML*, therapy-related AML; *del*, deletion of one allele; *3*, three fluorescence signals indicating the translocation breakpoint; *di*, disomy (two fluorescence signals indicating retention of both alleles)

the distal part of band 7q22 and band 7q31 and was defined by the MDS/AML cases (Fig. 1). The breakpoint of a reciprocal translocation t(3;7)(p13;q22) (case no. 6) was localized to a 400-kb genomic segment in 7q22 within the deletion cluster of the MDS/AML cases. The breakpoint of a second translocation t(3;7)(q28;q22) (case no. 25) was mapped to 7q21.3, which is centromeric to both of the commonly deleted regions.

Using the same technique, Le Beau et al. (1996) recently delineated a 2- to 3-Mb commonly deleted genomic segment in band 7q22 in 15 patients with myeloid or lymphoid malignancies. This segment is contained within the genomic region identified in our study. DNA markers common to both regions include *D7S658, D7S796, D7S818, D7S2504, D7S2509*, and *D7S2494* (Fig. 2). Interestingly, the breakpoint of the reciprocal translocation t(3;7)/(p13;q22) which we identified in our study (case no. 6) maps not only to the critical region of our MDS/AML cases but also to the smallest overlapping deleted segment identified in the study of Le Beau et al. (1996). In this case of MDS, the translocation was present in unstimulated bone marrow and phytohemagglutinin-stimulated blood, indicating that the rearrangement had occurred either in an early hematopoietic precursor cell differentiating to the myeloid or the lymphoid lineage, or in the germline, and then probably predisposed the patient to the development of MDS. This translocation breakpoint may point to a novel gene of pathogenetic significance in myeloid leukemias.

Johnson et al. (1996) reported on a family in which multiple members in a three-generation pedigree hat a constitutional inversion inv(7)(q22.1;q34). One individual of this family had developed MDS and another had pancytopenia. The proximal breakpoint of this constitutional inv(7) and the break-

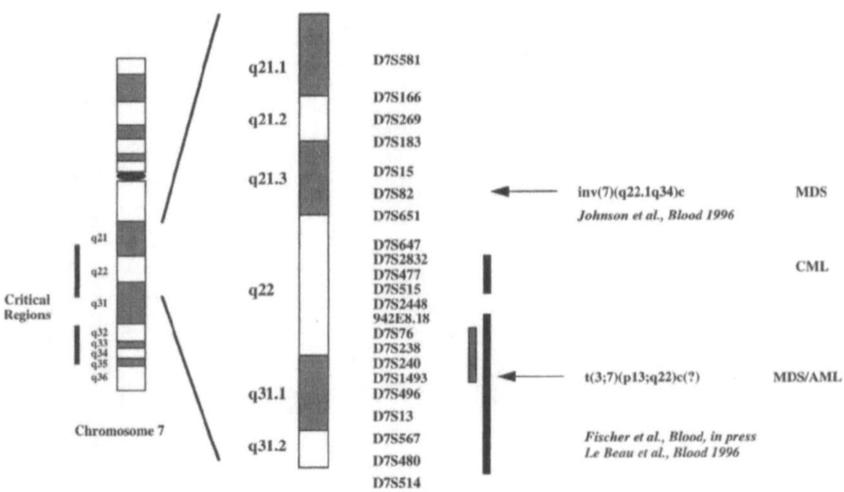

Fig. 2. Review of the studies which aimed at mapping aberrations of chromosome band 7q22 in malignant myeloid disorders using FISH

point of a reciprocal translocation t(2;7)(p13;q22) in an unrelated patient with MDS were found to be contained in a genomic fragment identified by a 650-kb-sized YAC clone. This region, which includes the gene for the cell-cycle control enzyme ASNS, maps proximal to the translocation breakpoint of our MDS patient and to the commonly deleted segments that were identified in our study (Fischer et al. 1997) and that of Le Beau et al. (1996) (Fig. 2). Therefore, it is unlikely that this genomic region contains a specific gene(s) that is important in the pathogenesis of the majority of MDS.

Conclusion

Taken together, these data show heterogeneity of 7q22 deletion and translocation/inversion breakpoints in myeloid leukemias. Nevertheless, a single genomic region at 7q22 seems to be affected in the majority of MDS and AML cases, probably containing a new tumor suppressor gene involved in the pathogenesis of malignant myeloid disorders. Once candidate genes from this critical region are identified, it will be necessary to analyze MDS/AML tumors associated with 7q22 deletions for mutations of the remaining allele. Furthermore, it will be of interest to screen for germline mutations of the relevant genes, to evaluate whether there are patients who are at risk of developing therapy-related myeloid disorders following chemo- and/or radiotherapy for a malignant disease.

Acknowledgments. This work is supported by grants from the Tumorzentrum Heidelberg/Mannheim and the Canadian Genome Analysis and Technology Program (CGAT).

References

Bloomfield CD, de la Chapelle A (1987) Chromosome abnormalities in acute nonlymphocytic leukemia: clinical and biological significance. Semin Oncol 14:372–383

Fischer K, Fröhling S, Scherer SW, McAllister Brown J, Scholl C, Stilgenbauer S, Tsui LC, Lichter P, Döhner H (1997) Molecular cytogenetic delineation of deletions and translocations involving chromosome band 7q22 in myeloid leukemias. Blood (in press)

Fourth International Workshop on Chromosomes in Leukemia 1982 (1984) Abnormalities of chromosome 7 resulting in monosomy 7 or in deletion of the long arm (7q-): review of translocations, breakpoints and associated abnormalities. Cancer Genet Cytogenet 11:300–303

Johansson B, Mertens F, Mitelman F (1993) Cytogenetic deletion maps of hematologic neoplasms: circumstantial evidence for tumor suppressor loci. Genes Chromosomes Cancer 8:205–218

Johnson EJ, Scherer SW, Osborne L, Tsui LC, Oscier D, Mould S, Cotter FE (1996) Molecular definition of a narrow interval at 7q22.1 associated with myelodysplasia. Blood 87:3579–3586

Kere J, Ruutu T, Davies KA, Roninson IB, Watkins PC, Winqvist R, de la Chapelle A (1989a) Chromosome 7 long arm deletion in myeloid disorders: a narrow breakpoint region in 7q22 defined by molecular mapping. Blood 73:230–234

Kere J, Donis-Keller H, Ruutu T, de la Chapelle A (1989b) Chromosome 7 long-arm deletions in myeloid disorders: terminal DNA sequences are commonly conversed and breakpoints vary. Cytogenet Cell Genet 50:226–229

Kunz J, Scherer SW, Klawitz I, Soder S, Du YZ, Speich N, Kalff-Suske M, Heng HHQ, Tsui LC, Grzeschik HK (1994) Regional localization of 725 human chromosome 7-specific yeast artificial chromosome clones. Genomics 22:439–448

Le Beau MM, Albain KS, Larson RA, Vardiman JW, Davis EM, Blough RR, Golomb HM, Rowley JD (1986) Clinical and cytogenetic correlations in 63 patients with therapy-related myelodysplastic syndromes and acute nonlymphocytic leukemia: further evidence for characteristic abnormalities of chromosomes nos. 5 and 7. J Clin Oncol 3:325–345

Le Beau MM, Espinosa R III, Davis EM, Eisenbart JD, Larson RA, Green ED (1996) Cytogenetic and molecular delineation of a region of chromosome 7 commonly deleted in malignant myeloid diseases. Blood 88:1930–1935

Lewis S, Abrahamson G, Boultwood J, Fidler C, Potter A, Wainscoat JS (1996) Molecular characterization of the 7q deletion in myeloid disorders. Br J Haematol 93:75–80

Luna-Fineman S, Shannon KM, Lange BJ (1995) Childhood monosomy 7: epidemiology, biology, and mechanistic implications. Blood 85:1985–1999

Mitelman F, Brandt L, Nilsson PG (1978) Relation among occupational exposure to potential mutagenic/carcinogenic agents, clinical findings, and bone marrow chromosomes in acute nonlymphocytic leukemia. Blood 52:1229–1237

Mitelman F, Kaneko Y, Berger R (1995) Report of the committee on chromosome changes in neoplasia. In: Cuticchia AJ, Pearson PL (eds) Human gene mapping. Johns Hopkins, Baltimore, MD, p 773

Rabbitts TH (1994) Chromosome translocation in human cancer. Nature 372:143–149

Rodrigues Pereira Velloso E, Michaux L, Ferrant A, Hernandez JM, Meeus P, Dierlamm J, Criel A, Louwagie A, Verhoef G, Boogaerts M, Michaux JL, Bosly A, Mecucci C, Van den Berghe H (1996) Deletions of the long arm of chromosome 7 in myeloid disorders: loss of band 7q32 implies worst prognosis. Br J Haematol 92:574–851

Scherer SW, Tompkins BJF, Tsui LC (1992) A human chromosome 7-specific genomic DNA library in yeast artificial chromosomes. Mammal Genome 3:179–181

Scherer SW, Poorkaj P, Trask B, Soder S, Allen T, Nunez M, Geshuri D, Wong E, Belloni E, Little S, Zhou L, Becker D, Kere J, Ignatius J, Niikawa N, Fukushima Y, Hasegawa T, Weissenbach J, Boncinelli E, Massa H, Tsui LC, Evans JP (1994) Physical mapping of the split hand/split foot locus *(SHFD1)* on chromosome 7 and implication in syndromic ectrocactyly. Hum Mol Genet 3:1345–1354

Tsui LC, Donis-Keller H, Grzeschik KH (1995) Report of the Second International Workshop on Human Chromosome 7 Mapping 1994. Cytogenet Cell Genet 71:1–34

Molecular Cytogenetic Analysis of Low-Grade B-Cell Neoplasias: a Comparative Genomic Hybridization Study

C.A. Werner[1], H. Döhner[1], T.F.E. Barth[2], S. Stilgenbauer[1], A. Plesch[1], P. Lichter[3], and M. Bentz[1]

[1] Department of Internal Medicine V, University of Heidelberg, Hospitalstraße 3, 69115 Heidelberg, Germany
[2] Institute of Pathology, University of Ulm, Germany
[3] German Cancer Research Center, Im Neuenheimer Feld 280, Heidelberg, Germany

Introduction

Malignant tumors are characterized by deregulation of cell proliferation and differentiation, often induced by genomic alterations within the tumor cells (see Fischer et al., this volume). In acute leukemias, chromosomal banding analyses have greatly contributed to our understanding of key mechanisms in leukemogenesis. One important example is the identification of protooncogenes, such as MLL, ETO, AML 1, or TEL, which are activated by recurrent chromosomal translocations. In addition, specific chromosomal aberrations are closely associated with the phenotype of the tumor cells and even clinical features such as response to therapy and the probability of long-term survival (Pui 1995).

Cytogenetic analysis of low-grade lymphoproliferative disorders has proven more difficult. In these diseases, chromosomal banding techniques are hampered by the limited availability of fresh tumor tissue and the restriction to metaphase cells, which may not be representative of the tumor cell population. In contrast, fluorescence in situ hybridization (FISH) using specific DNA probes has greatly improved the ability to detect chromosomal aberrations, since interphase nuclei can be analyzed (Bentz et al. 1994; Le Beau 1993). However, this technique depends on preknowledge of candidate regions and on the availability of suitable DNA probes. Furthermore, only a few genomic regions can be analyzed within a single FISH experiment.

Comparative genomic hybridization (CGH) is a method that allows rapid screening of chromosomal imbalances within tumor genomes without the need for specific probes (Kallioniemi et al. 1992). For CGH analysis, differentially labeled genomic tumor and control DNAs are cohybridized to normal metaphase chromosomes under suppression conditions and detected via different fluorochromes. Digitized image analysis is used to measure the fluorescence intensities of tumor and control DNA and to calculate fluorescence ratio values for each chromosome region. Thus, overrepresented and underrepresented DNA sequences can be mapped within the tumor genome (Lichter et al. 1995). So far, numerous CGH studies have been performed, the vast majority of which focussed on the analysis of solid tumors (Houldsworth and Chaganti

Recent Results in Cancer Research, Vol. 144

1994). In low-grade lymphoproliferative disorders, only a few CGH studies have been reported (Bentz et al. 1995b, 1996). In the following, results of studies in two different types of low-grade B-cell neoplasias, chronic B-cell lymphocytic leukemia (B-CLL) and follicle center lymphoma (FCL; Kiel classification: centroblastic-centrocytic non-Hodgkin's lymphoma), are summarized.

Chronic B-Cell Leukemias

B-CLL is the most prevalent leukemia in Europe and North America. Although banding analysis has revealed a number of recurrent chromosomal aberrations, little is known about the prognostic relevance of specific karyotype abnormalities. In banding studies, a complex karyotype was the only independent chromosome abnormality which was associated with an inferior outcome by multivariate analysis (Juliusson et al. 1990). The poor correlation of chromosomal banding data with the clinical course in B-CLL may be explained by technical problems in culturing B-CLL cells for cytogenetic analysis: the leukemic cells exhibit a low proliferative activity, and in about 50% of the cases no chromosomal abnormalities are detected (Juliusson et al. 1990). This is, at least in part, due to mitotic cells arising from nonleukemic T lymphocytes in the blood of B-CLL patients (Knuutila et al. 1986). Thus, molecular cytogenetic studies using CGH appeared to be a promising approach, because this technique does not rely on the preparation of metaphase spreads.

Using CGH, we analyzed 40 patients with chronic B cell leukemias [37 with B-CLL and three with B-cell prolymphocytic leukemia (B-PLL)]. The imbalances detected most frequently were losses of genetic material on chromosome arms 17p (nine cases), 11q (five cases), 13q (four cases), and 6q (three cases), and overrepresentations on 3q (four cases), 8q (three cases), 12q (six cases), 15q (two cases), and 17q (two cases). A synopsis of all abnormalities identified by CGH is shown in Fig. 1 (black symbols). Many of these imbalances are well known to occur in chronic B cell leukemias. However, gains of chromosomal material on the long arm of chromosome 8, which were detected in 3 of the 40 cases, have not been described as a recurrent aberration in these tumors before (Bentz et al. 1995b). In two of the three cases, the CGH findings were confirmed by FISH, whereas in the third case, no material was available for further analysis. All cases with overrepresentations on the chromosomal arm 8q were also examined by banding analysis, which in each case failed to detect this aberration.

Another new finding was the presence of highly amplified DNA sequences in three different chromosomal regions. Double minute chromosomes (dmins) or homogeneously staining regions (hsrs), the cytogenetic hallmarks of gene amplification, have been reported only sporadically in chronic B cell leukemias (Mitelman 1994). Due to the potential of CGH, the chromosomal map positions of the amplified sequences were readily identified (see Fig. 2): in one patient, two distinct amplification sites mapping to the short arm of

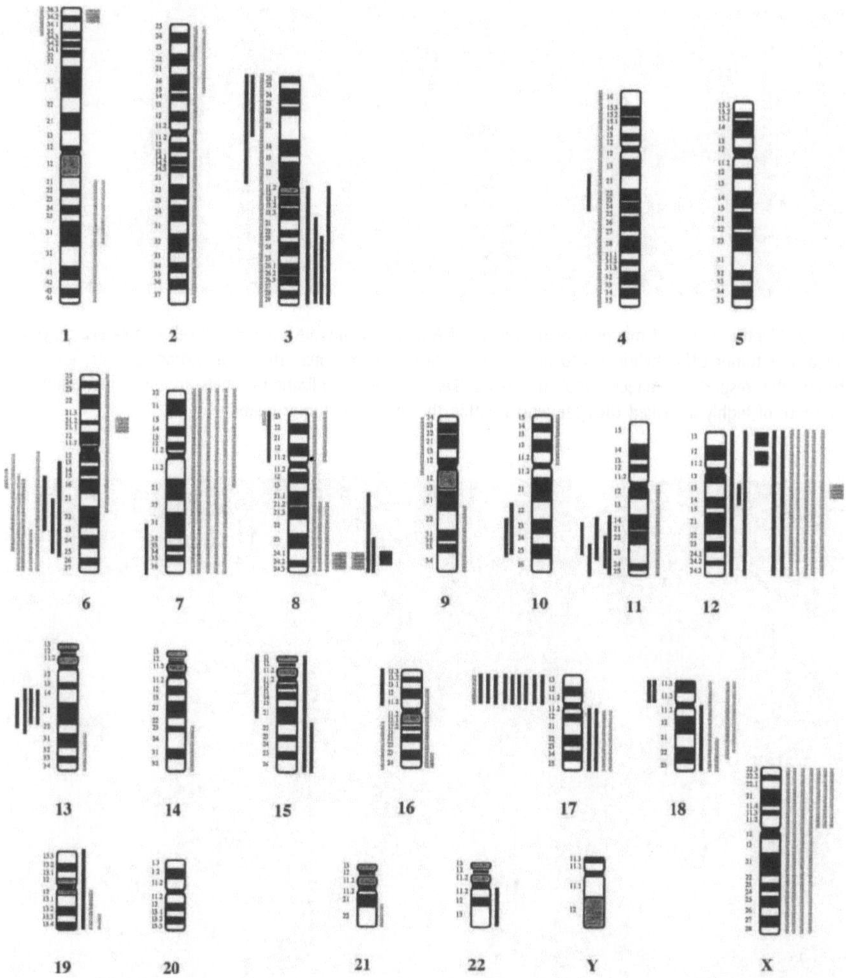

Fig. 1. Summary of chromosomal imbalances detected in 40 patients with chronic B-cell leukemia (*black symbols*) and 28 patients with follicle center lymphoma *gray symbols*). Lines on the *left side* of the ideograms indicate losses of chromosomal material; lines on the *right side* indicate gains of chromosomal sequences. *Squares* represent high-level DNA amplifications

chromosome 12 were present (12p11–12 and 12p13). In another patient, amplified sequences derived from the chromosomal band 8q24 were detected. This coincides with the localization of the *MYC* protooncogene, which plays a major role in other types of lymphoproliferative disorders. By FISH analysis using a *MYC*-specific cosmid probe an amplification was detected in 5% of the cells as a large, dispersed hybridization signal.

In 28 of the 40 patients, G-banding data were available. Comparison of these data with the CGH data showed a high proportion of cases (13 of 28),

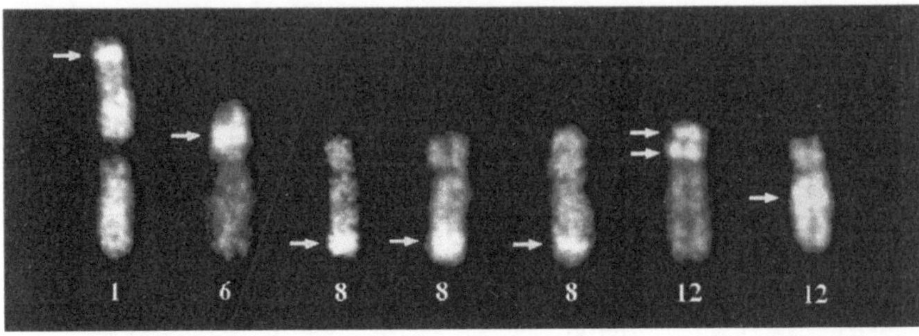

Fig. 2. Identification and mapping of high-level DNA amplifications in low-grade B-cell neoplasias: grayscale images of tumor DNAs hybridized to normal metaphase chromosomes. The chromosome numbers are given below the respective images. Note the band-like, intense hybridization signals (*arrows*) indicating the presence of highly amplified DNA sequences within the respective tumor genomes

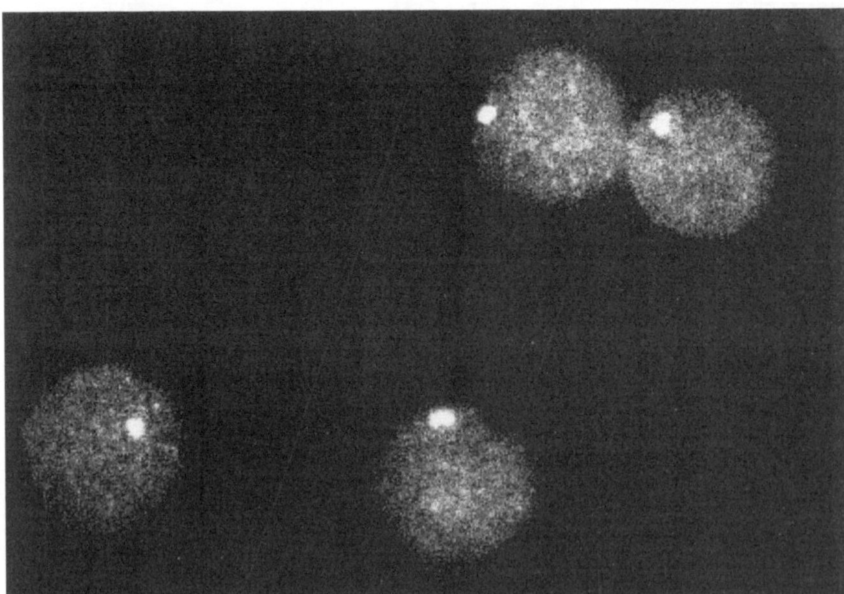

Fig. 3. Interphase cytogenetic analysis of a case with B-CLL using a yeast artificial chromosome probe mapping to band 11q23. Only one hybridization signal is visible in the cells, indicating a deletion on 11q23. On banding analysis, this case had a normal karyotype, whereas CGH, revealed a loss of chromosomal material on bands 11q22–25

where additional chromosomal imbalances were detected by CGH. In the majority of cases with such discrepancies, the CGH results were tested by FISH using specific DNA probes. In each of these cases, the CGH finding was confirmed (for an example, see Fig. 3). These data indicate that in a considerable proportion of CLL cases, additional abnormalities can be found by CGH.

This is particularly evident in cases which exhibited no karyotypic abnormalities by chromosomal banding analysis: in 6 of 13 cases with a normal karyotype on G-banding analysis, chromosomal imbalances were detected by CGH. Such discrepancies between chromosome changes present in the interphase cells but not in the proliferating cell fraction have been detected before in cases of trisomy 12 as well as deletions of 13q and 17p (Döhner et al. 1993, 1995); Stilgenbauer et al. 1993). In these FISH studies, higher incidences of the respective chromosomal aberrations were found than suspected by banding analysis.

The finding that, in a significant number of cases, CGH revealed chromosomal imbalances not detected by banding analysis implies that in cytogenetic studies relying on banding analysis in CLL, possibly relevant karyotype changes are missed in a considerable proportion of cases. In another study, we compared banding and CGH data in ten cases of myeloid leukemias without finding any discrepancies (Bentz et al. 1995a). This indicates that banding data in general reflect the chromosomal changes in the malignant clone in these disorders. This may explain why it was possible to identify specific chromosomal changes with a high prognostic impact in acute leukemias (Bloomfield and de la Chapelle 1987; Maurer et al. 1991), whereas in CLL such clinically important aberrations are still a matter of discussion.

The importance of these findings is underlined by two FISH studies identifying prognostically relevant genetic aberrations in chronic B-cell leukemias. Deletions of both the p53 gene and a chromosomal subregion mapping to band 11q23 identify subgroups of CLL patients with an inferior prognosis as demonstrated by multivariate analysis (Döhner et al. 1995, 1997).

Follicle Center Lymphomas

Follicle center lymphomas are characterized by the chromosomal translocation t(14;18)(q32;q21), which has been found in more than 80% of cases (Yunis et al. 1982). At the molecular level, this translocation juxtaposes the *BCL2* protooncogene located on chromosomal band 18q21 to regulatory sequences of the immunoglobulin heavy chain gene on band 14q32, resulting in enhanced *BCL2* expression. Although *BCL2* overexpression inhibits apoptosis, conferring a survival advantage to the t(14;18)-positive cells, its sole presence does not render the cells malignant, as demonstrated in a transgenic mouse model (for review see Korsmeyer 1992). This is confirmed by the finding of t(14;18)-positive cells in cases of benign lymphoid tissues with follicular hyperplasia and even in the peripheral blood of healthy donors (Limpens et al. 1991; Liu et al. 1994; Poetsch et al. 1996).

Thus, it is likely that additional genetic changes are crucial for the development of follicle center lymphoma. These may be submicroscopic (e.g., point mutations or microdeletions) and therefore not detectable by cytogenetic techniques. However, in the data bank of the Catalog of Chromosome Aberrations in Cancer (Mitelman 1994), 320 of 355 t(14;18)-positive lymphomas are recorded as exhibiting secondary chromosomal aberrations, especially microscopically detectable gains and losses of genetic material (Johansson et al. 1995). In view of this, CGH analysis of follicle center lymphoma appears a promising approach. Here, we summarize CGH data of 28 patients with the classical follicular variant of follicle center lymphoma. A *BCL 2/IgH* rearrangement was present in 25 out of the 28 patients (89%) as determined by polymerase chain reaction or interphase FISH. In 20 of the 28 patients, chromosomal imbalances were identified by CGH. The results are summarized in Fig. 1 (gray symbols). The most frequent aberrations were gains on chromosomes X (7 cases), 7 (6 cases), 8 (6 cases), 12 (6 cases), and 18 (4 cases), and losses on the long arm of chromosome 6 (6 cases). High-level DNA amplifications were identified in five instances on chromosomal bands 1p36, 6p21, 8q24 (two cases), and 12q13.

These findings are in agreement with banding data (Johansson et al. 1995). In addition, for chromosomes X, 8, 12, and 18, our CGH data allowed further narrowing of the relevant subregions which might harbor genes relevant for lymphoma progression. On chromosome X, the whole chromosome was overrepresented in four instances, while in three cases only the short arm was affected. On chromosome 12, a high-level DNA amplification mapping to bands 12q13–14 pinpointed a possible consensus region. This coincides with the localization of several protooncogenes such as *MDM2, ERBB3, GLI,* and *SAS* (OMIM 1996). On chromosome 18, the commonly overrepresented region mapped to bands 18q21–22, the locus of the *BCL2* protooncogene. A consensus region on the long arm of chromosome 8 was defined by the presence of highly amplified DNA sequences on band 8q24, which were observed in two cases.

In contrast to previous studies in non-Hodgkin's lymphoma (NHL) using other cytogenetic techniques, we identified a high incidence of high-level DNA amplifications (five amplifications in 4 of the 28 patients). DNA amplifications represent one of the mechanisms for upregulating the expression of genes. In malignancies, cellular oncogenes are often part of the amplified genomic regions. Amplification of cellular oncogenes has been found in many solid tumors. In several instances, an association with a more aggressive tumor phenotype and an inferior outcome has been established (Schwab and Amler 1990). By contrast, gene amplification has been considered a rare event in NHL. Using banding analysis, dmins and hsrs were identified in only 19 out of more than 3000 NHL cases (Mitelman 1994), and only few additional cases with amplifications have been identified by other techniques. CGH is particularly sensitive for the detection of high-level DNA amplifications because the high copy number difference between the amplified sequences (>5 to more than 100 copies) and normal chromosomal regions (two copies) allows reliable identification of amplicons as small as 100 kb (Joos et al. 1993). In addition, CGH has the advantage of mapping the amplified sequences within the genome, immediately pinpointing candidate genes extracted from the existing gene map. In this way, the identification of critical genes within the amplicons is greatly facilitated. The DNA amplifications of this series of 28 patients with follicle center lymphoma mapped to four different genomic regions; 1p36, 6p21, 8q24 (two cases), and 12q13–14. Band 8q24 is the chromosomal locus of the *MYC* protooncogene. A synergistic effect of *MYC* activation and *BCL2* deregulation was demonstrated in double transgenic mice (Strasser et al. 1990). These animals developed rapidly growing lymphomas with an immature phenotype. For this reason, *MYC* was further analyzed in both cases with an amplification mapping to 8q24. In both cases, an *MYC* amplification was demonstrated by Southern blot analysis. Together with the finding of a *MYC* amplification in a case with a chronic B-cell leukemia, these data suggest that *MYC* amplification is not a rare event in low-grade B-cell neoplasias. It is possible that activation of *MYC* via gene amplification may be a relevant mechanism in patients with gains of genetic material on chromosome 8.

In conclusion, CGH allows several technical problems to be overcome, that severely impaired cytogenetic studies in low-grade lymphoproliferative disorders. Chromosomal aberrations were identified in a high proportion of CLL cases with a normal banding karyotype. In addition, several chromosomal regions of possible pathogenetic relevance were delineated. Further molecular analyses will contribute to the elucidation of the clinical and biological relevance of specific chromosome aberrations in these tumors.

Acknowledgment. This work was supported by the Deutsche Forschungsgemeinschaft (grant Be 1454/5-1).

References

Bentz M, Döhner H, Cabot G, Lichter P (1994) Fluorescence in situ hybridization in leukemias: the FISH are spawning! Leukemia 8:1447–1452

Bentz M, Döhner H, Huck K, Schütz B, Ganser A, Joos S, du Manoir S, Lichter P (1995a) Comparative genomic hybridization in the investigation of myeloid leukemias. Genes Chromosomes Cancer 12:193–200

Bentz M, Huck K, du Manoir S, Joos S, Werner CA, Fischer K, Döhner H, Lichter P (1995b) Comparative genomic hybridization in chronich B-cell leukemias reveals a high incidence of chromosomal gains and losses. Blood 85:3610–3618

Bentz M, Werner CA, Döhner H, Joos S, Barth TFE, Siebert R, Schröder M, Stilgenbauer S, Fischer K, Möller P, Lichter P (1996) High incidence of chromosomal imbalances and gene amplifications in the classical follicular variant of follicle center lymphoma. Blood 88:1437–1444

Bloomfield CD, de la Chapelle A (1987) Chromosome abnormalities in acute nonlymphocytic leukemia: clinical and biological significance. Semin Oncol 14:372–383

Döhner H, Pohl S, Bulgay-Mörschel M, Stilgenbauer S, Bentz M, Lichter P (1993) Trisomy 12 in chronic lymphoid leukemias – a metaphase and interphase cytogenetic analysis. Leukemia 7:716–720

Döhner H, Fischer K, Bentz M, Hansen K, Cabot G, Benner A, Diehl D, Schlenk R, Coy J, Volkmann M, Galle PR, Poustka A, Hunstein W, Lichter P (1995) p53 gene deletion predicts for poor survival and non-response to therapy with purine analogs in chronic B-cell leukemias. Blood 85:1580–1589

Döhner H, Stilgenbauer S, James MR, Benner A, Bentz M, Fischer K, Hunstein W, Lichter P (1997) 11q deletions identify a new subset of B-cell chronic lymphocytic leukemia characterized by extensive nodal involvement and inferior prognosis. Blood (in press)

Houldswirth J, Chaganti RSK (1994) Comparative genomic hybridization: an overview. Am J Pathol 145:1253–1260
Johansson B, Mertens F, Mitelman F (1995) Cytogenetic evolution patterns in non-Hodgkin's lymphomas. Blood 86:3905–3914
Joos S, Scherthan H, Speicher MR, Schlegel J, Cremer T, Lichter P (1993) Detection of amplified genomic sequences by reverse chromosome painting using genomic tumor DNA as probe. Hum Genet 90:584–589
Juliusson G, Oscier DG, Fitchett M, Ross FM, Stockdill G, Mackie MJ, Parker AC, Castoldi GL, Cuneo A, Knuutila S, Elonen E, Gahrton G (1990) Prognostic subgroups in B-cell chronic lymphocytic leukemia defined by specific chromosomal abnormalities. N Engl J Med 323:720–724
Kallioniemi A, Kallioniemi O-P, Sudar D, Rutovitz D, Gray JW, Waldman F, Pinkel D (1992) Comparative genomic hybridization for molecular cytogenetic analysis of solid tumors. Science 258:818–821
Knuutila S, Elonen E, Teerenhovi L, Rossi L, Leskinen R, Bloomfield CD, de la Chappelle A (1986) Trisomy 1 2 in B-cell of patients with B-cell chronic lymphocytic leukemia. N Engl J Med 314:865–869
Korsmeyer SJ (1992) Bcl-2 initiates a new category of oncogenes: regulators of cell death. Blood 80:879–886
Le Beau MM (1993) Detecting genetic changes in human tumor cells: have scientists "gone fishing". Blood 81:1979–1983
Lichter P, Bentz M, Du Manoir S, Joos S (1995) Comparative genomic hybridization. In: Verma R, Babu A (eds) Human chromosomes. McGraw-Hill, New York, pp 191–210
Limpens J, de Jong D, van Krieken JHJM, Price CGA, Young BD, van Ommen GJB, Kluin PM (1991) *Bcl-2*/J_H rearrangement in benign lymphoid tissues with follicular hyperplasia. Oncogene 6:2271–2276
Liu Y, Hernandez AM, Shibata D, Cortopassi GA (1994) BCL2 translocation frequency rises with age in humans. Proc Natl Acad Sci USA 91:8910–8914
Maurer J, Janssen JWG, Thiel E, van Denderen J, Ludwig WD, Aydemir Ü, Heinze B, Fonatsch C, Harbott J, Reitter A, Riehm H, Hoelzer D, Bartram C (1991) Detection of chimeric BCR-ABL genes in acute lymphoblastic leukemia by the polymerase chain reaction. Lancet 337:1055–1058
Mitelman F (1994) Catalog of chromosome aberrations in cancer. Wiley Liss, New York
OMIM (1996) Online mendelian inheritance in man. Center for Medical Genetics, Johns Hopkins University, Baltimore MD, and National Center for Biotechnology Information, National Library of Medicine, Bethesda, MD
Poetsch M, Weber-Matthiesen K, Plendl H-J, Schlegelberger B (1996) Detection of the t(14;18) chromosomal translocation by interphase cytogenetics with YAC probes in follicular lymphoma and nonneoplastic lymphoproliferation. J Clin Oncol 14:963–969
Pui C-H (1995) Childhood leukemias. N Engl J Med 332:1618–1630
Schwab M, Amler L (1990) Amplification of cellular oncogenes: a predictor of clinical outcome in human cancer. Genes Chromosomes Cancer 1:181–193
Stilgenbauer S, Döhner H, Bulgay-Mörschel M, Weitz S, Bentz M, Lichter P (1993) High frequency of monoallelic retinoblastoma gene deletion in B-cell chronic lymphoid leukemia shown by interphase cytogenetics. Blood 81:2118–2124
Strasser A, Harris AW, Bath ML, Cory S (1990) Novel primitive lymphoid tumours induced in transgenic mice by cooperation between *myc* and *bcl-2*. Nature 348:331–333
Yunis YY, Oken MM, Kaplan ME, Ensrud KM, Howe RB, Theolgides A (1982) Distinctive chromosomal abnormalities in histologic subtypes of non-Hodgkin's lymphoma. N Engl J Med 307:1231–1236

Applications of Gene Transfer in Hematologic Malignancy

M. K. Brenner

Cell and Gene Therapy Program, St. Jude Children's Research Hospital,
332 N. Lauderdale, Memphis, TN 38105, USA

Abstract

Although gene transfer was originally conceived as a means to replace or correct defective genes in patients with inherited disorders, the process has shown broad potential for intervention in hematologic malignancy and for study of hematopoietic stem cell biology.

Gene transfer strategies now under investigation for these applications include

1) repair of one or more genetic defects associated with the malignant process,
2) delivery of a prodrug-metabolizing enzyme that causes tumor cells to become sensitive to the corresponding anticancer drug,
3) modification of immune responses to the cancer, and
4) introduction of drug resistance genes to increase the therapeutic index of cytotoxic agents.

Finally, by marking normal or malignant cells with readily detectable genes, one can monitor the efficacy of therapy or study the dynamics of stem cell behavior in vivo.

At present these applications are limited by the quality of vectors, but as transduction efficiencies and gene regulatory mechanisms improve, gene transfer can be expected to evolve into a major therapeutic modality in its own right.

Introduction

Strategies for incorporating gene transfer into cancer treatment protocols are varied but in general entail modifying the tumor cell itself, either by "repairing" one or more of the genetic defects associated with the malignant process, by introducing a gene that will trigger an antitumor immune response, or by delivering a prodrug-metabolizing enzyme that will render the tumor sensitive to the corresponding cytotoxic agent. One can also modify

Recent Results in Cancer Research, Vol. 144

immune responses to the tumor, by altering the specificity or effector function of immune system cells, or decrease the sensitivity of normal host tissue with drug resistance genes, thereby increasing the therapeutic index of cytotoxic agents. Finally, by marking normal or malignant cells with easily tracked genes, one can monitor the efficacy of conventional treatments. Examples of each of these applications follows.

Correction of Specific Genetic Defects

The most attractive approach to treating hematologic neoplasia by gene transfer would be to correct the specific genetic lesions that increasingly are being shown to contribute to the malignant phenotype. Unfortunately, unless the inserted gene is lethal to the cell, the progeny will likely harbor additional defective genes that will render the cell effectively premalignant, with a high risk of later transformation. Moreover, many defective genes produce molecules with "transdominant" effects that will perpetuate the malignant phenotype even when a wild-type gene is introduced, requiring their neutralization by methods that are not yet fully evolved (antisense RNA, ribozymes, or homologous recombination with a wild-type gene) (Snyder et al. 1993; Scanlon et al. 1991; Ratajczak et al. 1992). Moreover, success can only be achieved if a very high proportion of the cells are successfully transduced – an outcome that is simply not yet possible, since leukemia and lymphoma cells are known to be resistant to transduction by most available vectors (Table 1). Hence it may be difficult for the tumor cell correction approach to eradicate a clonal malignancy (Anderson 1990; Rossi 1995).

Several groups have nonetheless taken the position that certain genetic abnormalities are more essential to cancer induction and progression than others, and are attempting to neutralize fusion transcripts, such as *BCR-ABL* (Snyder et al. 1993), or activated oncogenes, such as *MYB* (Ratajczak et al. 1992) or *K-RAS* (Zhang et al. 1993), using ribozymes, antisense RNA, or wild-type genes (see Kronenwett and Haas, this volume, and James, this volume). There are also plans to restore nonfunctional antioncogenes, such as *p53*, as well as genetic programs that regulate apoptosis (Fujiwara et al. 1993; Wang et al. 1995). Preliminary work in animal model systems indicates that even minor perturbations in cell regulatory pathways can significantly modify the sensitivity of cells to chemotherapy.

Conversion of Prodrugs into Lethal Cytotoxins

Another potentially useful strategy now under investigation is the transfer of genes that encode enzymes able to convert harmless prodrugs into lethal cytotoxins (Ramet et al. 1993; see also Günzburg et al., this volume). To selectively kill malignant hematopoietic cells, either the gene vector or the activity of the (pro)drug must be specifically targeted. Early attempts to achieve

Table 1. Vectors used in hematologic malignancy

Vectors	Advantages	Disadvantages
Retroviruses	1. Wide target cell range 2. Integrate in host DNA, so long-term expression in dividing cells 3. Nontoxic in absence of helper viruses	1. Only infect cells in cycle – therefore unusable for many hematologic diseases 2. Low efficiency of transfer even in susceptible cells 3. Too unstable for in vivo use
Adenoviruses	1. Wide target cell range in general 2. Infect nondividing cells 3. Stable in vivo	1. Poor infection in many lymphoid and some myeloid malignancies 2. Transient expression since nonintegrating 3. Highly immunogenic/inflammatory
Adeno-associated virus	1. Non-toxic (apparently) 2. Integrate in host DNA (??site-specific) 3. Wide target cell range and appear stable in vivo	1. Very high numbers of particles needed for infection/integration 2. May require adenovirus products for efficient transduction – difficult to manufacture in bulk 3. Limited size of inserted gene
Liposomes	1. Nontoxic and can be given repeatedly 2. Inherently noninfectious, so safety issues less troubling	1. Low efficiency of transfer 2. Unstable in vivo 3. Transient expression

this result (in solid tumors) made use of retroviral vectors to introduce a thymidine kinase-gene into tumor cells (Ram et al. 1993). On exposure to ganciclovir, the transduced cells should phosphorylate the drug. If the cell then divides, the product will be incorporated into DNA with lethal consequences, without affecting nondividing cells. Although initial reports of the efficacy of this approach (in primary and secondary brain tumors) were encouraging, the immediate likelihood of similar successes in hematologic cancers is low, owing to the difficulty or specifically targeting and transducing hematopoietic cells. If, however, the technology for gene transfer improves, there will be more than a dozen prodrug systems available for use. Of these, cytosine deaminase (which converts 5-fluorocytosine to 5-fluorouracil), P450-2B1 (which converts cyclophosphamide to 4-hydroperoxycyclophosphamide) (Wei et al. 1994) and the bacterial nitroreductase system (which reduces CB 1954 to the more active 4-hydroxylamine) (Knox et al. 1993) are perhaps the most attractive for therapeutic applications.

Modification of the Immune System

A considerable body of evidence indicates that the immune system has the potential to eradicate hematologic malignancy. This effect is most apparent in patients who have received bone marrow allografts, in whom graft-versus-host disease (GvHD) appears to reduce the risk of subsequent relapse, while T-cell depletion or other anti-GvHD measures are associated with an increased risk of disease recurrence (Horowitz et al. 1990). This so-called graft-versus-leukemia (GvL) effect may simply be another manifestation of GvHD, in which both normal and malignant host cells share the same host-specific polymorphism that are targets for alloreactive T lymphocytes. On the other hand, T cells that react with tumors cells may be recognizing discrete target antigens. Hematologic malignancies may express a number of tumor-specific proteins such as immunoglobulin or T-cell receptor idiotypes, mutated oncoproteins and fusion proteins generated by chromosomal translocation or viral proteins. If these proteins are processed to peptides and presented on the cell surface in association with major histocompatibility complex (MHC) molecules, they may induce a potent, malignancy-specific, T-cell-mediated response (Brenner and Heslop 1991; Nelief and Kast 1993; see chapter 9). Two general proposals have been made to exploit these sources of immunogenicity. One relies on gene transfer to modify the malignant cell to make it more immunogenic, while the second utilizes infusion of tumor-specific cytotoxic T cells prepared ex vivo. In the latter strategy, gene transfer effectively enhances the effector cell function.

Tumor Cell Immunogens

Some investigators are attempting to strengthen immune response against weakly immunogenic tumors by transducing tumor cells with cytokine genes (Brenner and Heslop 1991; Melief and Kast 1993; Nabel et al. 1993; Chen et al. 1992; Townsend and Allison 1993; Tepper et al. 1989; Golumbek et al. 1991; Fearow et al. 1990; Gansbacher et al. 1990; Colombo et al. 1991; Colombo and Forni 1994) with allogeneic MHC molecules (Nabel et al. 1993) or with B7.1 (Chen et al. 1992; Townsend and Allison 1993) a costimulatory molecule that activates cytotoxic T cells after engaging their surface CD28 or CTLA4 ligands (see Meuer et al., this volume). In murine models, the injection of such transduced neoplastic cells in doses that would have normally caused a tumor instead recruited immune system effector cells and eradicated injected tumor cells, as well as established tumors at distant sites. These results have important implications for the treatment of hematologic malignancy, as they suggest that one can overcome the barriers of imprecise targeting and inefficient transduction in vivo by transducing a small number of cells ex vivo and using them to immunize the patient.

The concept of tumor cell immunogens is being evaluated in more than 40 different clinical trials, mostly in solid tumor patients. Preliminary findings in melanoma, renal cell carcinoma, and neuroblastoma suggest that tumor cells transduced with HLA-B7, GM-CSF, or IL-2 can be given safely and will often produce objective immunomodulatory effects, including peripheral blood eosinophilia, a rise in the number and activity of natural killer or activated killer cells, and the generation of tumor-specific T cells (Nabel et al.

1993; Gansbacher et al. 1990; Colombo and Forni 1994). In several patients, these effects have translated into antitumor responses. These are encouraging results and suggest a role for the approach as adjuvant therapy for prevention of relapse in patients with suspected minimal residual disease. Efforts are now being made to maximize immune responses by inserting several different immunostimulatory genes into tumor cells. The feasibility of this approach has been demonstrated in preclinical studies of lymphotactin and IL-2, in which a combination of this T cell chemokine and a T cell growth factor caused regressions of established leukemias that were resistant to either agent alone (Dilloo et al. 1997).

Gene-Modified Cytotoxic T Cells

Lymphoproliferative disease due to Epstein-Barr virus (EBV) affords a useful model with which to evaluate the antitumor effects of gene-modified cytotoxic T lymphocytes (CTL) in patients (Papadopoulos et al. 1994; Rooney et al. 1995). Although EBV-infected B cells are highly immunogenic and normally susceptible to killing by specific CTL, in immunocompromised patients they may grow unchecked, producing a rapidly progressive lymphoproliferative disease that usually appears histologically as an immunoblastic lymphoma. This complication occurs in 1%–30% of patients receiving immunosuppressive therapy after allografting and is fatal in a high percentage of this subgroup. This, if EBV-infected cells are able to flourish because of the absence of functional, EBV-reactive CTL, administration of normal peripheral blood lymphocytes from EBV-immune donors to patients with lymphoproliferative disease should be curative. In fact, administration of donor peripheral blood mononuclear cells to recipients after marrow allografting has produced complete clinical and histological responses, presumably due to virus-specific T cells within the bulk lymphocyte population (Papadopoulos et al. 1994). However, since such cell populations also contain many alloreactive T cells, the treatment may induce severe GvHD.

An attractive alternative is the use of T cells specific only for the viral antigens expressed by the tumor cells. In one study, EBV-specific CTL lines were adoptively transferred to patients after marrow allografting to assess the safety and efficacy of this treatment again EBV-immunoblastic lymphoma (Rooney et al. 1995). Since the T cells were first marked with the neomycin resistance gene (*neo*^{R}) before they were injected, it was also possible to determine the cells distribution pattern, longevity, and antitumor activity in vivo. In the first 25 patients treated, the infused CTL had no adverse effects and were long-lived, since *neo*^{R}-bearing lymphocytes were detected at postinfusion intervals as long as 18 months. In four patients with evidence of EBV reactivation, CTL therapy was associated with a 1000-fold decrease in EBV-DNA levels in peripheral blood within 3–4 weeks after infusion. In two striking cases, the treatment eliminated biopsy-proven immunoblastic lymphomas.

Enhanced Production of Cytotoxic Cytokines

It may also be possible to enhance the antitumor activity of lymphocytes by increasing the levels of cytotoxic cytokines they produce at local tumor sites (Rosenberg 1992; see also Günzberg, this volume). This strategy, which is being evaluated in studies with tumor-infiltrating lymphocytes (TILs), has several inherent difficulties, one being that TILs resist attempts to elicit increased production of cytokines. Nonetheless, a sustained response was noted in one of the first six patients whose TILs secreted transgenic tumor necrosis factor.

Modification of Drug Sensitivity

If normal hemopoietic stem cells could be rendered resistant to one or more cytotoxic drugs, it might be possible to circumvent the myelosuppressive effects of cancer chemotherapy, so that treatment can be extended or intensified, perhaps with improved clinical outcome (Murphy et al. 1993; Levin and Hryniuk 1987). Hence, the *MDR1* gene has been widely considered for human therapy (see Fruehauf et al., this volume). The *MDR 1* product, P-glycoprotein, functions as a drug efflux pump, conferring resistance to many antineoplastic drugs. Experiments with murine models support the idea that the *MDR 1* transgene will protect hematopoietic cells from chemotherapy (Pastan and Gottesman 1991; Mickisch et al. 1991 a, b; McLachlin et al. 1990). Currently, three clinical trials are testing whether transfer of the *MDR 1* gene to bone marrow or peripheral blood stem cells from adult cancer patients will attenuate the myelosuppressive effects of chemotherapy. Other drug resistance genes that may afford therapeutic opportunities include those encoding DNA-methylguanine methyltransferases (MGMTs), enzymes that repair DNA damage product by the nitrosoureas, a class of alkylating agents used widely in cancer chemotherapy (Moritz et al. 1993). Preliminary data suggest that retrovirally mediated transfer of the human *MGMT* gene to mouse bone marrow cells will protect murine progenitor cells from the toxic effects of BCNU. Genes specifying dihydrofolate reductase and topoisomerase II are also under consideration for clinical testing.

The prospects for successful clinical application of drug resistance gene transfer are clouded by several considerations. First of all, the low stem cell transduction efficiencies observed with current clinical protocols predict that amelioration of drug-induced myelosuppression will not occur unless in vivo cell selection is substantial. There is also the risk that transfer of drug resistance genes to tumor cells will contaminate the marrow graft and produce drug-resistant relapse. Finally, toxicity to nonprotected organs, including gut, heart, and lungs, may nullify the gains secured from induction of marrow resistance.

Genetic Marking of Hematopoietic Stem Cells

Genetic marking of hematopoietic cells allows us to gain insight into patterns of cell survival, localization, and function. This approach has been used to determine the origin of relapse in patients undergoing autologous hematopoietic stem cell rescue for acute myeloid leukemia (AML) and neuroblastoma. Such information is critical because disease recurrence could arise from malignant cells introduced into the patient, suggesting the need for more effective purging (Brenner et al. 1993; Rill et al. 1994).

Thus, using retroviral vectors, we genetically marked the bone marrow of 12 patients who were scheduled to receive autologous bone marrow transplants from AML. Of the four patients who relapsed, three had cells bearing the marker gene. The specificity of this finding was reinforced by the presence of cells (in one case) positive for the neo^R gene and coexpressing the CD34 and CD56 antigens, a combination not found on normal hematopoietic cells. These cells also displayed *AML1/ETO* fusion transcripts that could be identified by the polymerase chain reaction (Brenner et al. 1993). Similar results have been obtained by M.D. Anderson investigators in adult patients undergoing autologous marrow transplantation for chronic myeloid leukemia (Deisseroth et al. 1994).

Taken together, these results demonstrate that bone marrow harvested from patients in apparent clinical remission may contain residual tumorigenic cells and that these cells can contribute to disease recurrence, indicating that more effective purging techniques will be needed to improve the outcome of autologous transplantation procedures - a goal that could be aided by the use of two distinctive genetic markers to distinguish between purged and unpurged cells. Double gene marking is also being used to determine which combinations of cytokines are more likely to induce long-term repopulating marrow cells to divide, leading to shorter periods of marrow hypoplasia after transplantation.

Conclusion

Gene transfer studies have made valuable contributions to extant and emerging knowledge concerning the genetic treatment of hematologic cancers. As the quality of vector technology improves, we can expect to see gene transfer evolve into a therapeutic modality in its own right.

Acknowledgments. Some of the work described in this article was supported by NIH grant CA 20180, Cancer Center Support CORE grant CA 21765, and the American Lebanese Syrian Associated Charities (ALSAC). We wish to thank Genetic Therapy, Inc., for providing the clinical grade vectors described in the section on gene marking, and Nancy Parnell for word processing.

References

Anderson WF (1990) The ADA human gene therapy clinical protocol. Hum Gene Ther 1:327–362

Brenner MK, Heslop HE (1991) Graft-versus-host reactions and bone marrow transplantation. Curr Opin Immunol 3:752–757

Brenner MK, Rill DR, Moen RC et al (1993) Gene-marking to trace origin of relapse after autologous bone marrow transplantation. Lancet 341:85–86

Chen L, Ashe S, Brady WA et al (1992) Costimulation of antitumor immunity by the B7 counterreceptor for the T lymphocyte molecules CD28 and CTLA-4. Cell 71:1093–1102

Colombo MP, Forni G (1994) Cytokine gene transfer in tumor inhibition and tumor therapy: where are we now? Immunol Today 15:48–51

Colombo MP, Ferrari G, Stoppacciaro A et al (1991) Granulocyte colony-stimulating factor gene transfer suppresses tumorogenicity of a murine adenocarcinoma in vivo. J Exp Med 173:889–897

Deisseroth AB, Zu Z, Claxton D et al (1994) Genetic marking shows that Ph+ cells present in autologous transplants of chronic myelogenous leukemia (CML) contribute to relapse after autologous bone marrow transplantation in CML. Blood 83:3068–3076

Dilloo D, Bacon K, Holden W et al (1997) Chemokine and cytokine gene transfer enhances antitumor immunity. Nature Med (in press)

Fearon ER, Pardoe DM, Itaya T et al (1990) Interleukin-2 production by tumor cells bypasses T helper function in the generation of an antitumor response. Cell 60:397–403

Fujiwara T, Grimm EA, Cai DW, Owen-Schaub LB, Roth JA (1993) A retroviral wild-type p53 expression vector penetrates human lung cancer spheroids and inhibits growth by inducing apoptosis. Cancer Res 53:4129–4133

Gansbacher B, Zier K, Daniels B, Cronin K, Bannerji R, Gilboa E (1990) Interleukin-2 gene transfer into tumor cells abrogates tumorigenicity and induces protective immunity. J Exp Med 172:1217–1224

Golumbek PT, Lazenby AJ, Levitsky HI et al (1991) Treatment of established renal cancer by tumor cells engineered to secrete interleukin-4. Science 254:713–716

Horowitz MM, Gale RP, Sondel PM et al (1990) Graft-versus-leukemia reactions after bone marrow transplantation. Blood 75:555–562

Knox RJ, Friedlos F, Boland MP (1993) The bioactivation of CB 1954 and its use as a prodrug in antibody-directed enzyme prodrug therapy (ADEPT). Cancer Metastasis Rev 12:195–212

Levin L, Hryniuk WM (1987) Dose intensity analysis of chemotherapy regimens in ovarian carcinoma. J Clin Oncol 5:756

McLachlin JR, Eglitis MA, Ueda K et al (1990) Expression of a human complementary DNA for the multidrug resistance gene in murine hematopoietic precursor cells with the use of retroviral gene transfer. J Natl Cancer Inst 82:1260

Melief CJ, Kast WM (1993) Potential immunogenicity of oncogene and tumor suppressor gene products. Curr Opin Immunol 5:709–713

Mickisch GH, Licht T, Merlino GT, Gottesman MM, Pastan I (1991a) Chemotherapy and chemosensitization of transgenic mice which express the human multidrug resistance gene in bone marrow: efficacy, potency, and toxicity. Cancer Res 51:5417

Mickisch GH, Merlino GT, Galski H, Gottesman MM, Pastan I (1991b) Transgenic mice that express the human multidrug-resistance gene in bone marrow enable a rapid identification of agents that reverse drug resistance. Proc Natl Acad Sci USA 88:547

Moritz T, Mackay W, Feng LJ, Samson L, Williams DA (1993) Gene transfer of O^6-methylguanine methyltransferase (MGMT) protects hematopoietic cells (HC) from nitrosourea (NU)-induced toxicity in vitro and in vivo (Abstr). Blood 82 Suppl 1:118a

Murphy D, Crowther D, Renninson J et al (1993) A randomised does intensity study in ovarian carcinoma comparing chemotherapy given at four week intervals for six cycles with half dose chemotherapy given for twelve cycles. Ann Oncol 4:377

Nabel GJ, Nabel EG, Yang ZY et al (1993) Direct gene transfer with DNA-liposome complexes in melanoma: expression, biologic activity, and lack of toxicity in humans. Proc Natl Acad Sci USA 90(23):11307–11311

Papadopoulos EB, Ladanyi M, Emanuel D et al (1994) Infusions of donor leukocytes to treat Epstein-Barr virus-associated lymphoproliferative disorders after allogeneic bone marrow transplantation. N Engl J Med 330:1185–1191

Pastan I, Gottesman MM (1991) Multidrug resistance. Annu Rev Med 42:277

Ram Z, Culver KW, Walbridge S et al (1993) In situ retroviral-mediated gene transfer for the treatment of brain tumors in rats. Cancer Res 83–88

Ratajczak MZ, Kant JA, Luger SM et al (1992) In vivo treatment of human leukemia in a SCID mouse model with c-myb antisense oligodeoxynucleotides. Proc Natl Acad Sci USA 89:11823–11827

Rill DR, Santana VM, Roberts WM et al (1994) Direct demonstration that autologous bone marrow transplantation for solid tumors can return a multiplicity of tumorigenic cells. Blood 84:380–383

Rooney CM, Smith CA, Ng C et al (1995) Use of gene-modified virus-specific T lymphocytes to control Epstein-Barr virus-related lymphoproliferation. Lancet 345:9–13

Rosenberg SA (1992) Gene therapy for cancer. JAMA 268:2416–2419

Rossi JJ (1995) Therapeutic antisense and ribozymes. Br Med Bull 51:217–225

Scanlon KJ, Jiao L, Funato T et al (1991) Ribozyme-mediated cleavage of *c-fos* mRNA reduces gene expression of DNA synthesis enzymes and metallothionein. Proc Natl Acad Sci USA 88:10591–10595

Snyder DS, Wu Y, Wang JL et al (1993) Ribozyme-mediated inhibition of *bcr-abl* gene expression in Philadelphia chromosome-positive cell line. Blood 82:600–605

Tepper RI, Pattengale PK, Leder P (1989) Murine interleukin-4 displays potent anti-tumor activity in vivo. Cell 57:503–512

Townsend SE, Allison JP (1993) Tumor rejection after direct costimulation of CD8+ T cells by B7-transfected melanoma cells. Science 259:368–370

Wang J, Bucana CD, Roth JA, Zhang W (1995) Apoptosis induced in human osteosarcoma cells is one of the mechanisms for the cytocidal effect of Ad5CMV-p53. Cancer Gene Ther 2:9–18

Wei MX, Tamiya T, Chase M et al (1994) Experimental tumor therapy in mice using the cyclophosphamide-activating cytochrome P450 2B1 gene. Hum Gene Ther 5:969–978

Zhang Y, Mukhopadhyay T, Donehower LA, Georges RN, Roth JA (1993) Retroviral vector-mediated transduction of K-*ras* antisense RNA into human lung cancer cells inhibits expression of the malignant phenotype. Hum Gene Ther 4:451–460

Dendritic Cells for Somatic Gene Therapy

J. Westermann, A. Aicher, and A. Pezzutto

Department of Hematology/Oncology and Tumor Immunology,
Robert Rössle Clinic, Virchow Hospital, Humboldt University,
Lindenbergerweg 80, 13122 Berlin, Germany

Introduction

The identification of tumor-specific antigens in the last few years provides the basis for novel, specific immunotherapeutic strategies, since these antigens are potential targets for MHC-I-restricted CD8+ cytotoxic lymphocytes which mediate tumor rejection in animal models (Boon et al. 1994; Greenberg 1991). Antigens so far defined as being truly tumor-specific can be divided into different categories: mutated proteins such as k-ras, p53, or erb-b2, fusion proteins, which are gene products of chromosomal translocations, e.g., bcr/abl (p210) in chronic myeloid leukemia, idiotypic determinants of immunoglobulins, or T-cell receptors in lymphoid malignancies. Furthermore, shared antigens such as MAGE, which are expressed by melanoma and several other tumors but not in normal tissues (except testis), and differentiation antigens such as MelanA/Mart1 and tyrosine in melanoma, can serve as targets for immunotherapy.

The expression of the whole antigen on the cell surface is not essential to elicit a T-cell-mediated immune response. In recent years it has been demonstrated that both endogenous and exogenous proteins are delivered to the cell's antigen processing and presentation machinery. Intracellular proteins are degraded by the proteasome into small peptides 8–12 amino acids in length which are transported into the endoplasmic reticulum (ER) by TAP (transporter associated with antigen processing). In the ER, peptides are loaded into the binding groove of MHC class I molecules. The binding motif of each peptide contains anchor positions which determine the affinity to a given MHC-I molecule. If a peptide fits in the groove of a specific MHC-I molecule, the MHC-I-peptide complex is exported to the cell surface, where it can be recognized by CD8+ T-cells (reviewed in Rock 1996).

Failure of Immune Surveillance

If tumor-specific antigens are processed and presented to T cells, why can tumors grow in immunocompetent individuals? Although this question has not

Recent Results in Cancer Research, Vol. 144

been finally clarified, three basic mechanisms which enable the tumor to evade immunosurveillance have been elucidated: (a) defective antigen processing/presentation (e.g., downregulation of MHC-I, defects in the antigen processing machinery), (b) downmodulation of local T-cell activity (e.g., by cytokines such as transforming-growth-factor-β or IL-10, both produced in tumor tissue), and (c) lack of costimulation, leading to anergy (reviewed in Blankenstein et al. 1996; see also Meuer et al., this volume). Lack of costimulation seems to play a central role in tolerance towards tumor cells and relies on the observed fact that T cells require two signals for activation: antigen recognition in context with MHC molecules and costimulation by accessory molecules of the B7-family (B7.1 = CD80 or B7.2 = CD86) (Chen et al. 1992, 1993). Antigen presentation without concomitant costimulatory signal not only fails to active T cells; it can induce tolerance towards a particular antigen. In normal cells this mechanism may protect the organism from autoimmunity; in cancer cells it can provide a way of evading the immune response despite appropriate presentation of a tumor-specific antigenic epitope. In animal models it has been demonstrated that introduction of costimulatory molecules in tumor cells by means of gene transfer can restore immunogenicity and elicit antitumor responses (Townsend and Allison 1993; Chen et al. 1994).

A further approach to overcome tolerizing effects on tumor cells is the introduction of tumor-associated antigens into professional antigen-presenting cells (APC) such as dendritic cells (DC).

Dendritic Cells: Possible Use in Cancer Immunotherapy

DC play a pivotal role in the elicitation of an antigen-specific, MHC-restricted T-cell response and are thought to be the only APC able to prime naive T-cells (Steinman 1991). Nonfollicular DC are cells originating in the bone marrow which belong to the myeloid lineage. DC are located at high density near barriers to the outside world (skin, mucosa) and in the cellular interstitium. In their immature stage (Langerhans cell phenotype) they can capture antigens from their environment before starting migration into the T-cell areas of lymphoid tissues, where maturation is completed. The mature DC (interdigitating phenotype) is characterized by a low antigen uptake ability but high antigen presentation capacity. Antigens which have been taken up during this maturation process are presented to T cells in lymphoid tissue.

DC can be derived both from non-T/non-B peripheral blood mononuclear cells (PBMC) (Romani et al. 1994) and from CD34+ stem cells (Caux et al. 1992; Siena et al. 1995) by ex vivo cultivation in the presence of cytokines (Fig. 2). For clinical applications, DC can be generated from the monocytoid cell fraction after counterflow elutriation of PBMC and culture in the presence of GM-CSF and IL-4. By this method large numbers (10^9–10^{10}) of functionally active DC can be obtained. In particular, it appears that IL-4 is able to inhibit the differentiation of monocytes while turning them into DC (Peters et al. 1996). These monocyte-derived DC are functionally active.

The therapeutic application of ex-vivo-generated DC generally aims at inducing a cytotoxic T-cell response by loading DC with tumor-specific antigens, based on two strategies:

1. Transduction of genes coding for tumor-specific antigens in DC
2. Peptide pulsing of ex-vivo-generated DC using a tumor-specific antigen.

Recent data demonstrate that exogenous antigens can also enter the class I pathway of antigen presentation in DC and elicit a cytotoxic T-cell response. In animal models it was demonstrated that tumor antigen-pulsed DC are able to induce protective T-cell immunity against a subsequent tumor challenge and also against small tumors that are already established (Celluzzi et al. 1996; Paglia et al. 1996; Mayordomo et al. 1995; Zitvogel et al. 1996). The question whether gene-modified or antigen (peptide)-pulsed DC are more efficient as a vaccine will have to be addressed in preclinical models.

Apart from transducing tumor antigens into DC, there is another strategy of gene modification: transfer of genes coding for T-cell active cytokines. This approach aims at additionally amplifying the T-cell response to tumor antigens presented by DC. By analogy to vaccination with cytokine-transfected tumor cells, high local cytokine concentrations may perhaps be achieved. Ideally, these cytokine-secreting DC would only activate T cells that interact with their MHC-peptide complex. Figure 1 summarizes clinical vaccination strategies using DC.

DC Can be Generated from Different Sources

In our laboratory, DC were obtained from T-cell and B-cell-depleted PBMC after 7 days of cultivation in the presence of GM-CSF and IL-4 or from

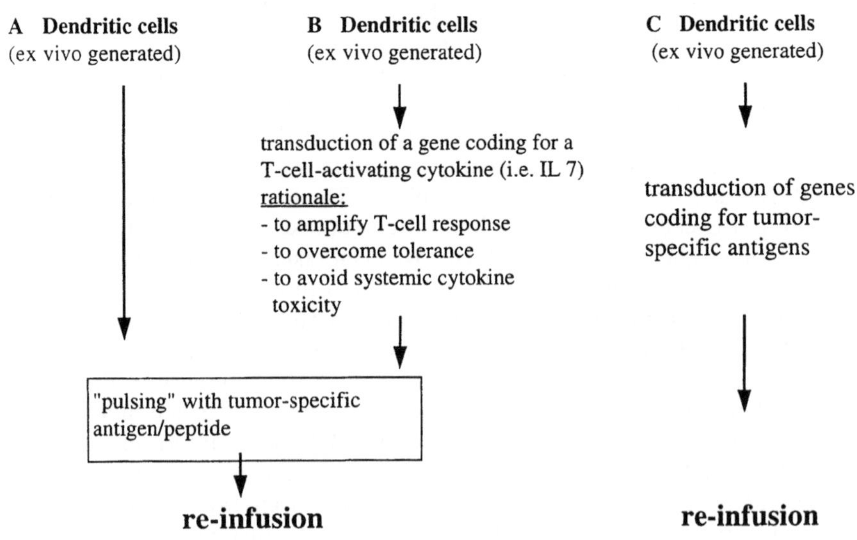

Fig. 1. Tumor vaccination studies using dendritic cells

CD 34+ stem cells after 12–14 days' cultivation with GM-CSF, TNFα, IL-4, and stem cell factor (SCF). The dendritic morphology of the cell populations was assessed by light and electron microscopy. On FACS analysis CD 3, CD 14, CD 16, and CD 19 antigens were negative. In contrast, MHC class-II molecules, CD 1 a, CD 80, CD 86, CD 40, CD 44, CD 54, and CD 4 were upregulated. The functional ability of DC was investigated by mixed lymphocyte reaction (MLR). Compared to PBMC and non-T-cells, DC showed an up to 30-fold stronger T-cell stimulation in allogeneic MLR and a 6- to 8-fold stronger stimulation in autologous MLR (Fig. 2).

Genetic Modification of DC

The feasibility of retroviral gene transfer into DC was demonstrated using the MFG vector with *lacZ* (coding for β-galactosidase) as a reporter gene. In various experiments a transfer efficiency of about 47% was achieved by repeated retroviral infection cycles, in particular at the beginning of the culture. Transfected DC still had high stimulatory capacity in MLR (Aicher et al. 1997).

In a series of further experiments, IL-7 was retrovirally transduced into DC for the following reasons: (a) to further amplify T-cell response and possibly break tolerance by high local cytokine concentrations, and (b) to augment CD 8+ T-cell recruitment (Alderson et al. 1990). Moreover, IL-7/B 7-co-transfected tumor cells induced strong T-cell activation and protective immunity in animal tumor models (Cayeux et al. 1995).

IL-7 gene transfer was performed using the retroviral vector pLXSN. In a series of four experiments transduced DC produced 3781±1926 pg IL-7/10^6 cells in 24 h. In allogeneic MLR an up to four-fold higher T-cell proliferation was achieved as compared to mock-transfected DC (Fig. 4).

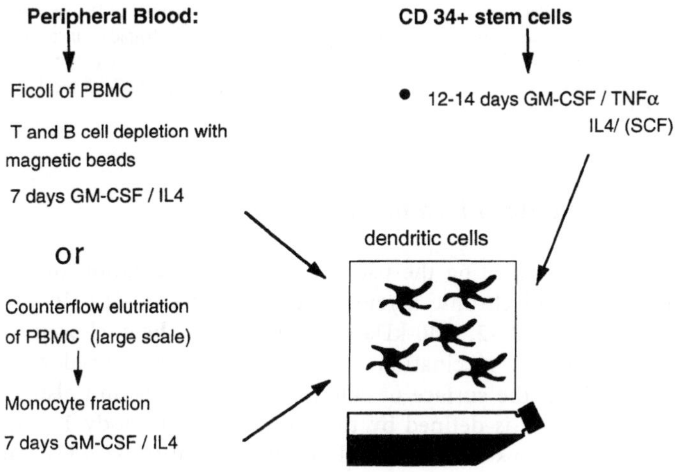

Fig. 2. Generation of dendritic cells

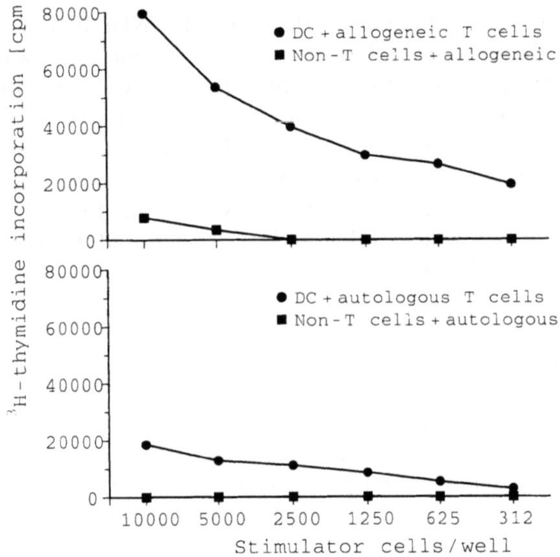

Fig. 3. Mixed lymphocyte reaction (MLR): T-cell proliferation measured in a ^{3}H-thymidine incorporation assay with different numbers of dendritic cells or non-T cells as stimulator cells and 10^5 autologous or allogeneic T cells. ^{3}H-thymidine incorporation (*vertical axis*) correlates to T-cell proliferation. *cpm* Counts per minute

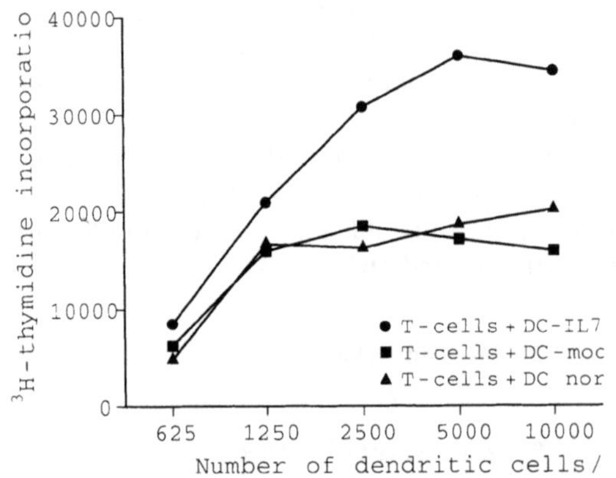

Fig. 4. Mixed lymphocyte reaction (MLR): T-cell proliferation measured in a ^{3}H-thymidine incorporation assay with 10^5 T cells and different numbers of unmodified, IL-7-transduced, and mock-transfected DC as stimulator cells. Horizontal axis shows the number of DC; vertical axis shows ^{3}H-thymidine incorporation (counts per minute, cpm) which correlates to T-cell proliferation

Clinical Models with Genetically Modified DC

As clinical models we are evaluating the use of DC-based vaccination in patients with colon cancer and chronic myelogenous leukemia (CML). In patients with colon cancer GA 733-2, a 40-kDa glycoprotein has been chosen as target molecule for DC-based vaccination. GA 733-2 is overexpressed as a type-I membrane protein at the surface of colon carcinoma cells and also in some other tumors. GA 733-2 is defined by the monoclonal antibody 17-1 A. Fagerberg et al. (1995) demonstrated a T-cell response against GA 733-2 in patients with colon cancer who were undergoing treatment with mAb 17-1 A.

Since T-cell epitopes of GA 733-2 have not yet been molecularly defined, it is necessary to use the whole antigen for vaccination strategies. Furthermore, this approach might promote induction of T-cell responses against multiple antigenic epitopes of the protein.

In our laboratory, the full-length variant GA 733-2-F and the truncated variant GA 733-2-E were amplified by reverse transcriptase polymerase chain reaction from the colon carcinoma line SW620. cDNA was then cloned into the retroviral expression vectors SF and LXSN. Transduction into DC is currently being performed. Transduced DC will be evaluated for their ability to induce a cytotoxic T-cell response. A clinical trial with DC, genetically modified to express GA 733-2, is planned in patients with colon cancer.

In CML, leukemic cells are Philadelphia-chromosome-positive in more than 90% of cases. The molecular correlate of the Philadelphia chromosome is a reciprocal chromosomal translocation between chromosomes 9 and 22. This event transposes the c-ABL protooncogene from chromosome 9 to the breakpoint cluster region (BCR) on chromosome 22, resulting in a new hybrid oncogene BCR/ABL which codes for a chimeric fusion protein (bcr/abl) with abnormal tyrosine kinase activity, turning normal hematopoietic progenitor cells into abnormally proliferating cells. The fusion region of bcr/abl can be regarded as a neoantigen whose expression is limited to the malignant cell clone. Since the breakpoints are remarkably constant, there are only two variants of the 210-kDa bcr/abl protein: bcr2/abl2 and bcr3/abl2. In the fusion region of the bcr3/abl2 protein four oligopeptides with intermediate or high affinity to the HLA haplotypes A3, A11, and B8 have been defined (Bocchia et al. 1995). Two of the peptides elicit a cytotoxic T-cell response to autologous and HLA-matched allogeneic leukemic cells in vitro (Bocchia et al. 1996; Greco et al. 1996).

In CML patients, DC are generated from CD34+ stem cells. Up to 60% of the cell preparations consist of DC as assessed by morphologic, immunophenotypic, and functional criteria. In the accelerated phase of the disease, most CD34+ cells bear the BCR/ABL translocation. By fluorescence in situ hybridization (FISH) we demonstrated that a large portion (>90%) of the CD34+-derived DC from patients with accelerated CML bear the BCR/ABL translocation (manuscript in preparation). These cells can be assumed to present bcr3/abl2 peptides to T cells. This situation makes CML particularly interesting as a clinical model, since there is no need for genetic modification or peptide loading in order to achieve presentation of the relevant tumor antigen in the MHC molecule. IL-7 gene transduction, however, could amplify specific T-cell response in these patients. In vivo a large burden of leukemia cells presenting bcr/abl peptides without costimulation is likely to have caused tolerance. Amplification of the T-cell response by IL-7-secreting DC might help to break this state of unresponsiveness towards leukemia cells. We have been successful in introducing the IL-7 gene in CD34-derived DC of CML-patients; an IL-7 production of about 3500 pg/10^6 cells in 24 h was achieved.

For the future, tumor vaccination strategies using DC could be of particular clinical value in the stage of minimal residual disease, i.e., after complete clinical response to (high-dose) chemotherapy. Recent clinical data in patients with follicular B-cell lymphoma who received autologous DC pulsed with idiotypic protein as tumor-specific antigen are encouraging and suggest that DC-based vaccination has therapeutic potential for the future.

References

Aicher A, Westermann J, Cayeux S, Daemen K, Willimsky G, Uckert W, Blankenstein T, Dörken B, Pezzutto A (1998) Successful retroviral transduction of a reporter gene in human dendritic cells: feasibility of therapy with gene-modified antigen presenting cells. Exp Hematol 25:39–44

Alderson MR, Sassenfeld HM, Widmer MB (1990) Interleukin 7 enhances cytolytic T lymphocyte generation and induces lymphokine-activated killer cells from human peripheral blood. J Exp Med 172:577–587

Blankenstein T, Cayeux S, Qin Z (1997) Genetic cancer vaccines. Rev Physiol Biochem Pharmacol 129:3–49

Bocchia M, Wentworth PA, Southwood S, Sidney J, McGraw K, Scheinberg DA, Sette A (1995) Specific binding of leukemia oncogene fusion protein peptides to HLA class I molecules. Blood 85:2680–2684

Bocchia M, Korontsvit Z, Xu Q, Mackinnon S, Yang SY, Sette A, Scheinberg DA (1996) Specific human cellular immunity to bcr-abl oncogene-derived peptides. Blood 87:3587–3592

Boon T, Cerottini JC, Van den Eynde B, van der Bruggen P, Van Pel A (1994) Tumor antigens recognized by T lymphocytes. Annu Rev Immunol 12:337–365

Caux C, Dezutter-Dambuyant C, Schmitt D, Banchereau J (1992) GM-CSF and TNF-α cooperate in the generation of dendritic Langerhans cells. Nature 360:258–261

Cayeux S, Beck C, Aicher A, Dörken B, Blankenstein T (1995) Tumor cells cotransfected with interleukin-7 and B7-1 genes induce CD25 and CD28 on tumorinfiltrating T lymphocytes and are strong vaccines. Eur J Immunol 25:2325–2331

Celluzzi CM, Mayordomo JI, Storkus WJ, Lotze MT, Falo LD Jr (1996) Peptide-pulsed dendritic cells induce antigen-specific, CTL-mediated protective tumor immunity. J Exp Med 183:283–287

Chen L, Ashe S, Brady WA, Hellström I, Hellström KE, Ledbetter JA, McGowan P, Linsley P (1992) Costimulation of antitumor immunity by the B7 counterreceptor for the T lymphocyte molecules CD28 and CTLA-4. Cell 71:1093–1099

Chen L, Linsley PS, Hellström KE (1993) Costimulation of T cells for tumor immunity. Immunol Today 14:483–486

Chen L, McGowan P, Ashe S, Johnston JV, Hellström I, Hellström KE (1994) B7-1/CD80 transduced tumor cells elicit better systemic immunity than wild-type tumor cells admixed with *Corynebacterium parvum*. Cancer Res 54:5420–5428

Fagerberg J, Hjelm AL, Ragnhammar P, Frödin JE, Wigzell H, Mellstedt H (1995) Tumor regression in monoclonal antibody-treated patients correlates with the presence of anti-idiotype-reactive T lymphocytes. Cancer Res 55:1824–1827

Greco G, Fruci D, Accapezzato D, Barnaba V, Nisini R, Alimena G, Montefusco E, Vigneti E, Butler R, Tanigaki N, Tosi R (1996) Two bcr-abl junction peptides bind HLA-AB molecules and allow specific induction of human cytotoxic T lymphocytes. Leukemia 10:693–699

Greenberg PD (1991) Adoptive T cell therapy of tumors: mechanisms operative in the recognition and elimination of tumor cells. Adv Immunol 49:281–355

Hsu FJ, Benike C, Fagnoni F, Liles TM, Czerwinski D, Taidi B, Engelman EG, Levy R (1996) Vaccination of patients with B-cell lymphoma using autologous antigen-pulsed dendritic cells. Nature Med 2:52–58

Mayordomo JI, Zorina T, Storkus WJ, Zitvogel L, Celluzzi C, Falo LD, Melief CJ, Ilstad ST, Kast WM, Deleo AB, Lotze MT (1995) Bone marrow-derived dendritic cells pulsed with synthetic tumour peptides elicit protective and therapeutic antitumour immunity. Nature Med 1:1297–1302

Paglia P, Chiodoni C, Rodolfo M, Colombo MP (1996) Murine dendritic cells loaded in vitro with soluble protein prime cytotoxic T lymphocytes against tumor antigen in vivo. J Exp Med 183:317–322

Peters JH, Gieseler R, Thiele B, Steinbach F (1996) Dendritic cells: from ontogenetic orphans to myelomonocytic descendants. Immunol Today 17:273–278

Rock KL (1996) A new foreign policy: MHC class I molecules monitor the outside world. Immunol Today 17:131–137

Romani N, Gruner S, Brang D, Kämpgen E, Lenz A, Trockenbacher B, Konwalinka G, Fritsch PO, Steinman RM, Schuler G (1994) Proliferating dendritic cell progenitors in human blood. J Exp Med 180:83–93

Schendel D, Gansbacher B, Oberneder R, Kriegmair M, Hofstetter A, Riethmüller G, Segurado OG (1993) Tumor-specific lysis of human renal cell carcinomas by tumor-infiltrating lymphocytes. I. HLA-A2-restricted recognition of autologous and allogeneic tumor lines. J Immunol 151:4209–4220

Siena S, Di Nicola M, Bregni M, Mortarini R, Anichini A, Lombardi L, Ravagnani F, Parmiani G, Gianni A (1995) Massive ex vivo generation of functional dendritic cells from mobilized CD34+ blood progenitors for anticancer therapy. Exp Hematol 23:1463–1471

Steinman RM (1991) The dendritic cell system and its role in immunogenicity. Annu Rev Immunol 9:271–296

Townsend SE, Allison JP (1993) Tumor rejection after direct costimulation of CD8+ cells by B7-transfected melanoma cells. Science 259:368–371

Zitvogel L, Mayordomo JI, Tjandrawan T, DeLeo AB, Clarke MR, Lotze MT, Storkus WJ (1996) Therapy of murine tumors with tumor peptide-pulsed dendritic cells: dependence on T cells, B7 costimulation, and T helper cell 1-associated cytokines. J Exp Med 183:87–97

Construction of Immunogenic Tumor Cell Surfaces by Somatic Gene Transfer

S.C. Meuer[1], B. Gückel[2], M. Lindauer[3], W. Rudy, and U. Moebius[3]

[1] Institute for Immunology, Im Neuenheimer Feld 305, 69120 Heidelberg, Germany
[2] University Women's Hospital, Vossstrasse 7, 69115 Heidelberg, Germany
[3] German Cancer Research Center, Im Neuenheimer Feld 280, 69120 Heidelberg, Germany

Introduction

A contemporary model of T-lymphocyte activation (two-signal hypothesis) strongly suggests that in addition to recognition of peptide/MHC and, thus, tumor antigens by the T-cell antigen receptor, costimulatory signals are required for optimal T-cell clonal expansion and their differentiation into effector cells (Mueller et al. 1989; Schwartz 1990). Receptors for costimulatory signals have been identified and defined, among which CD2, CD11/18, CD28, CD4, and CD8 appear to play important roles. Their respective ligands/coreceptors are CD58, CD54, CD80/CD86, MHC II, and MHC I, respectively.

Tumor antigens which associate with MHC molecules and, therefore, potentially stimulate tumor responses can be derived from tumor-associated viruses, from products of genes that are specifically mutated in tumor cells, or from unaltered proteins that are overexpressed (Altmann et al. 1992; Gedde-Dahl et al. 1993; van der Bruggen 1991). Antigens derived from intracellular proteins of human tumors that are recognized by T lymphocytes have been identified at the molecular level in the case of melanoma (Traversari et al. 1992; Brichard et al. 1993; Kawakami et al. 1994a, b; Wölfel et al. 1995).

Tumor cells generally do not express MHC class-II molecules, and, in addition, their expression of costimulatory/accessory receptors is reduced or even completely absent. Moreover, some ligands of accessory receptors are naturally expressed in a tissue-specific manner. For example, CD80, which only exists in lymphoid tissue, is not normally found on epithelial cells (Freeman et al. 1989). Acitve downregulation of accessory molecules such as CD54 and CD58 and of MHC class-I molecules, respectively, has been postulated to contribute to immune escape (Smith et al. 1989; Pantel et al. 1991). Since tumor cells, for this reason, cannot deliver appropriate costimulatory signals, there is an explanation why, despite the presence of recognizable antigens, tumor cells cannot stimulate an immune response but rather induce a state of specific tolerance, thereby mimicking a natural mechanism of tolerance induction toward self (Mueller et al. 1989; Schwartz 1990).

Expression of genes encoding cytokines or costimulatory molecules in tumor cells is one way to circumvent the observed defects. In this regard, expres-

Recent Results in Cancer Research, Vol. 144

sion of interleukin (IL)-2, IL-4, interferon (IFN)-γ, tumor necrosis factor (TNF)-α, granulocyte/macrophage colony-stimulating factor, and also CD80 have been shown to induce tumor rejection in murine tumor models (Fearon et al. 1990; Tepper et al. 1989; Gansbacher et al. 1990; Blankenstein 1991; Dranoff et al. 1993; Chen et al. 1992; Townsend and Allison 1993). These approaches represent promising new developments towards enhancing immune reactions against human tumors (see Westermann et al. Günzburg et al., this volume).

Here we have investigated the capacity of representative tumor cell lines (breast cancer, ovarian cancer, colon cancer, melanoma) to induce primary immune responses of allogeneic T lymphocytes prepared from the peripheral blood of healthy donors. Because T-cell activation does not occur when wild-type tumor cells are employed in these studies, we have, in addition, evaluated the effects of transfecting the CD80 gene into such cells and compared this measure with a popular mode of tumor cell modification, namely addition of Newcastle disease virus (Bohle et al. 1990).

Methods, Results, and Discussion

To examine the expression of ligands for accessory receptors on a series of tumor cell lines, tumor cells were propagated in vitro and subsequently incubated with monoclonal antibodies directed at common determinants of human MHC I and MHC II molecules, as well as with antibodies directed at CD54, CD58, and the CD80 glycoproteins. Cell surface densities were quantitated employing indirect immunofluorescence and flow cytometry. As demonstrated, in all cases the expression of "adhesion molecules" and MHC gene products on tumor cells was strongly reduced as compared to the EBV-transformed lymphoblastoid cell line, EB2, which was employed as a control. The results shown in Fig. 1 are representative of a large number of cell lines of different derivations that were analyzed in our laboratory. Thus, it seems that a fundamental defect for stimulating immune responses exists at the level of costimulation due to impaired expression of ligands for T-cell accessory receptors.

One would anticipate that reconstitution of immune responsiveness at the level of cell-cell interaction (induction) should lead to the generation of a wide variety of cytokines of the T-cell population which per se is not deficient. Theoretically, this approach should be more "physiologic" than the expression of individual cytokine genes, which may reconstitute lymphocyte proliferation but not necessarily a balanced differentiative immune response in which a number of cytokine activities cooperate (Fig. 2).

When individual tumor cell lines were employed to stimulate T cells from the peripheral blood mononuclear population of healthy individuals, no signs of activation could be detected (Fig. 3). In contrast, B-lymphoblastoid cells (B-LCL) stimulate a vigorous proliferative response in vitro. Given the crucial contribution of costimulatory signals to the immune response and the results shown in Fig. 1, this finding is not surprising.

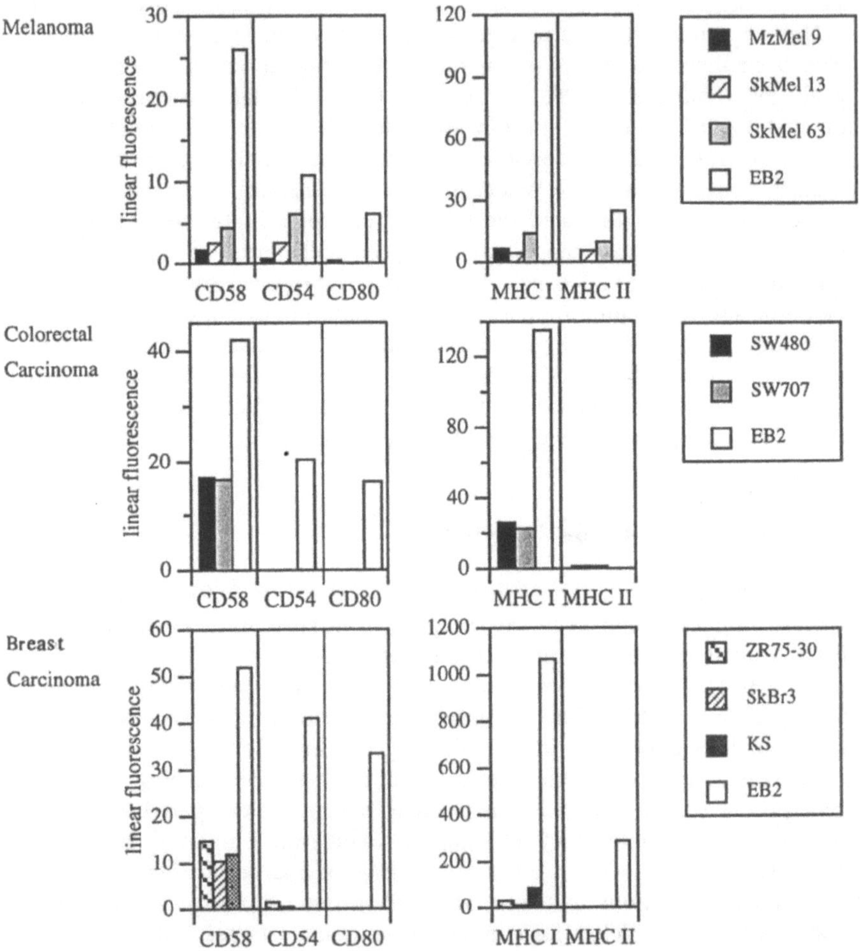

Fig. 1. Phenotypic analysis of tumor cell lines. Tumor cell lines were analyzed by indirect immunofluorescence using monoclonal antibodies as indicated at saturating concentrations together with a fluorescein-labeled secondary antibodies. Cell-bound fluorescence was evaluated by flow cytometry. Fluorescence intensity is given in linear arbitrary units

Expression of CD80, the ligand of the CD28/CTLA4 receptor of human T cells, by antigen-presenting cells has been shown to be critical for lymphocyte costimulation and for the prevention of T-cell anergy (Gimmi et al. 1993). Therefore, we investigated whether expression of CD80 through transfection of a plasmid containing the CD80 cDNA would represent an approach to enhance significantly the capacity of tumor cells to stimulate T-cell responses. Stable transfectants were established with a surface density of CD80 comparable to that found on B-LCLs (not shown). This was true for all four tumor types shown. Expression was stable for at least 6 months in

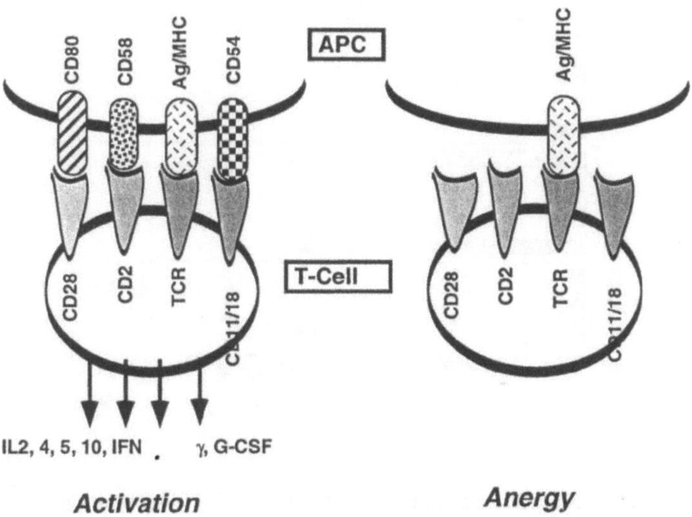

Fig. 2 Model of T-lymphocyte activation versus anergy induction by tumor cells. Antigen-presenting cells (*APC, lefthand side*) present antigen/MHC in association with ligands for T-cell coreceptors. This results in effective T-cell activation and, thus, in the release of cytokines which amplify the immune response. In the absence of costimulatory molecules (*righthand side*), as found in the case of tumor cells, antigen recognition leads to the induction of specific anergy

culture. Expression of the MHC molecules and CD54 and CD58 did not change when compared with non-transfected wild-type cells (not shown).

CD80 transfectants were subsequently examined regarding their potential to activate allogeneic T cells in vitro. As shown in Fig. 3, expression of CD80 on the representative melanoma and breast cancer cell lines showed a marked effect, i.e., reconstitution of T-cell proliferation. In contrast, in the case of colon carcinoma and ovarian carcinoma this was clearly not the case. This result suggest that CD80 appears to be required for T-cell costimulation but is not itself sufficient as an individual costimulus.

The effect of transfecting the CD80 plasmid into tumor cells was then compared with the effect of infecting cells with Newcastle disease virus (NDV), a popular approach in active specific immunotherapy (Bohle et al. 1990). Under these experimental conditions, at least, NDV infection of wild-type tumor cells did not show any detectable effect (Fig. 3). In contrast, in the case of CD80-transfected melanoma cells, NDV enhanced T-cell stimulation.

Previous investigation had demonstrated that cytokines, particularly TNF-α and IFN-γ, are capable of augmenting/upregulating the expression, not only of MHC class-I and class-II molecules, but also of CD54 and CD58 (Schirren et al. 1992). When we investigated the effects of pretreatment of wild-type breast and ovarian cancer cell lines with TNF-α and/or IFN-γ, we found that such a treatment upregulated the expression of MHC class I, MHC class II, and CD54, but not CD58. The combination of both cytokines induced even higher levels of CD54. In the case of CD80-transfected T-cell

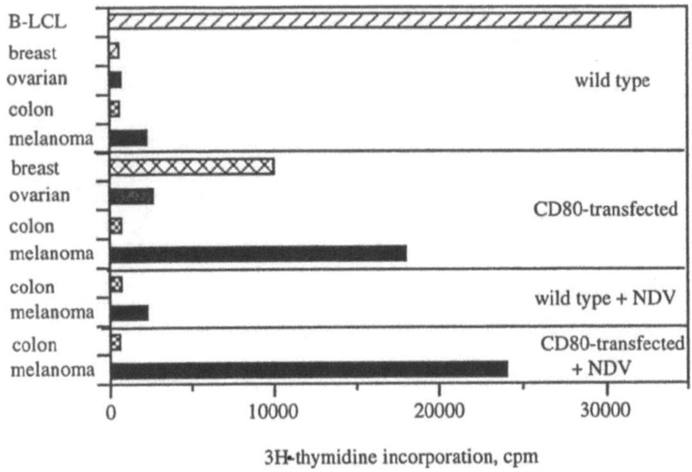

Fig. 3. T-cell proliferation induced by modified tumor cells. 10^5 T lymphocytes from healthy donors were stimulated with 10^4 irradiated allogeneic tumor cells for 5 days. T-cell proliferation was determined by 3 H-thymidine incorporation during the following 18 h incubation. Tumor cells used were either unmodified (wild-type), CD80-transfected, and/or NDV-infected. The following established tumor cell lines were used: KS (breast), GG (ovarian), SW480 (colon), SkMe 163 (melanoma), EBV-transformed B lymphoblasts (B-LCL). NDV infection was performed as described (Bohle et al. 1990). Stable CD80 transfectants are described elsewere (Gückel et al. 1995; Habicht et al. 1995)

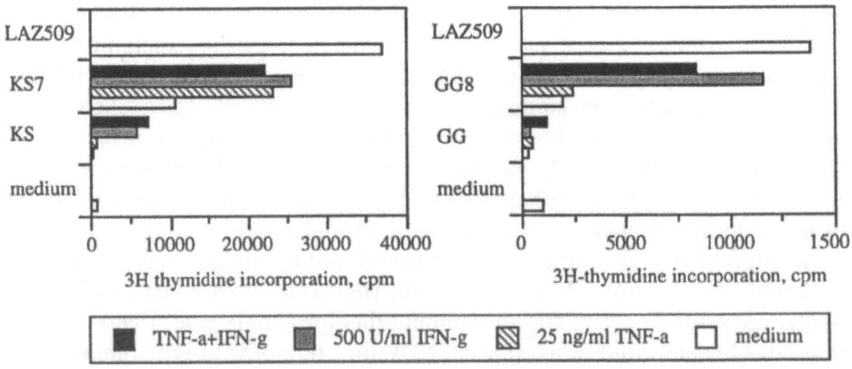

Fig. 4. Effect of cytokines on T-cell activation. 10^5 T cells were stimulated with 10^4 breast (KS) and ovarian tumor cells (GG), respectively. KS7 and GG8 are CD80-transfected variants of KS and GG, respectively. LAZ 509 is a EBV-transformed B-lymphoblastoid cell line. Tumor cells were used stimulator cells following pretreatment for 48 h with medium (*open bars*), TNF-α (*stripped bars*), INF-γ (*shaded bars*), or a combination of both cytokines (*solid bars*). Proliferative response of allogeneic T lymphocytes in the presence of 10 U/ml IL-2 was determined by 3 H-thymidine incorporation as in Fig. 3

clones, expression of CD 80 was slightly increased. Figure 4 shows the effects of cytokine pretreatment on tumor-cell-induced T-lymphocyte proliferation. Breast cancer cells (KS) preincubated with INF-γ, TNF-α, or a combination of both cytokines stimulated a proliferative response of T lymphocytes, whereas untreated cells did not. CD 80-expressing breast cancer cells (KS 7) were as effective as cytokine-preincubated parental KS cells. However, the combination of IFN-γ or TNF-α preincubation and CD 80 expression on KS cells resulted in an increased proliferation which was six-fold higher than that observed with cytokine-preincubated untransfected KS cells.

In the case of the ovarian cancer cells (GG), results were slightly different. Cytokine pretreatment of GG cells or, alternatively, transfection of CD 80 did not itself result in significant T-cell proliferation (compare Fig. 3). However, the preincubation of CD 80-positive GG 8 cells with IFN-γ or a combination of IFN-γ and TNF-α resulted in T cell activation. TNF-α alone had no effect on GG 8-induced T-cell proliferation, which goes along with the lack of effect on the cell surface density of CD 54 and MHC molecules (data not shown). Similar results to those shown in Fig. 4 were obtained with a series of additional CD 80-transfected KS and GG sublines excluding to a large extent clonal heterogeneity among transfected and nontransfected cells. In all cases, the T-cell proliferation promoted by CD 80 transfectants was specifically inhibited by CD 80 monoclonal antibodies.

Apparently, CD 80 cooperates with CD 54 in the induction of T-cell proliferation. This may explain the difference observed between the breast cancer cells KS, in which IFN-γ pretreatment augumented CD 54 expression, and the ovarian cancer cell line GG, where IFN-γ clearly had no effect on CD 54 cell surface expression. We have most recently obtained very similar information by studying a colon cancer cell line that was transfected and cotransfected with a number of different genes.

Although the data are not shown, while it is virtually impossible to generate T-cell lines employing wild-type tumor cells (even in the presence of cytokines such as IL-2), we have been able to propagate over considerable time periods (up to 100 days so far) T cells employing CD 80-transfected immunostimulatory cells, e.g., the breast cancer cell line KS 24 (Gückel et al. 1995). The proportion of activated ($CD25^+$)$CD8^+$ T-cells increased from 37% on day 25 to 71% on day 95. Importantly, these T lymphocytes were capable of killing unmodified KS cells (although CD 80-transfected KS cells were more effectively killed than wild-type cells, indicating that CD 80 plays a role not only in T-cell priming but also during the effector phase of cell-mediated lympholysis). Moreover, T-cell reactivity against KS tumor cells was MHC-restricted as taken from blocking studies employing MHC class I and CD 8 specific monoclonal antibodies. In contrast, antibodies directed at MHC class II or CD 4 did not exert inhibition (data not shown). The generation of MHC class I restricted CD 8 positive effector cells was only observed when CD 80 transfectants were employed for stimulation. In marked contrast, employing wild-type tumor cells and IL-2 in vitro generated predominantly LAK cells which could not be propagated long term (Gückel et al. 1995).

In conclusion, it appears that it is possible to reconstitute a fundamental defect in tumor cell/pre-effector cell interaction by transfecting particular genes encoding for ligands of accessory receptors required for costimulation of T lymphocytes. Employing this approach it is possible to generate class I restricted $CD8^+$ cytolytic effector T cells. The latter can be employed for the identification of novel tumor antigens in cancer types that have so far been considered nonimmunogenic (such as colon or ovarian cancer). Moreover, cancer cell lines transfected with adhesion molecules and enhanced immunogenicity may also serve as appropriate vaccines for the induction of tumor-specific immune response in vivo.

References

Altmann A, Jochmus-Kudielka I, Frank R, Gausepohl H, Moebius U, Gissmann L, Meuer SC (1992) Definition of immunogenic determinants of the human paillomavirus type 16 nucleoprotein E7. Eur J Cancer 28:326–333

Blankenstein T, Qin Z, Überla K, Müller W, Rosen H, Volk H-D, Diamantstein T (1991) Tumor suppression after tumor cell-targeted tumor necrosis factor-α gene transfer. J Exp Med 173:1047–1052

Bohle W, Schlag P, Liebrich W, Hohenberger P, Manasterski M, Möller P, Schirmacher V (1990) Postoperative active specific immunization in colorectal cancer patients with virus-modified autologous tumor-cell vaccine. Cancer 66:1517–1523

Brichard V, Van Pel A, Wölfel T, Wölfel C, De Plaen E, Lethe B, Coulie P, Boon T (1993) The tyrosinase gene codes for an antigen recognized by autologous cytolytic T lymphocytes on HLA-A2 melanomas. J Exp Med 178:489–495

Chen L, Ashe S, Brady WA, Hellström I, Hellström KE, Ledbetter JA, McGowan P, Linsley PS (1992) Costimulation of antitumor immunity by the B7 counterreceptor for the T lymphocyte molecule CD28 and CTLA-4. Cell 71:1093–1102

Dranoff G, Jaffee E, Lazenby A, Golumbek P, Levitsky H, Brose K, Jackson V, Hamada H, Pardoll D, Mulligan RC (1993) Vaccination with irradiated tumor cells engineered to secrete murine granulocyte-macrophage colony-stimulating factor stimulates potent, specific, and long-lasting antitumor immunity. Proc Natl Acad Sci USA 90:3539–3543

Fearon ER, Pardoll DM, Itaya T, Golumbeck P, Levitzky HI, Simons JW, Karasuyama H, Vogelstein B, Frost P (1990) Interleukin-2 production by tumor cells bypasses T helper function in the generation of an antitumor response. Cell 60:397–403

Freeman GJ, Freedman AS, Segil JM, Lee G, Whitman JF, Nadler LM (1989) B7, a member of the Ig superfamily with unique expression on activated and neoplastic B cells. J Immunol 143:2714–2722

Gansbacher B, Bannerji R, Daniels B, Zier K, Cronin K, Gilboa E (1990) Retroviral vector-mediated γ-interferon gene transfer into tumor cell generates potent and longlasting antitumor immunity. Cancer Res 50:7820–7825

Gedde-Dahl T III, Fossum B, Eriksen JA, Thorsby E, Gaudernack G (1993) T cell clones specific for p21 ras-derived peptides: characterization of their fine specificity and HLA restriction. Eur J Immunol 23:754–760

Gimmi CD, Freeman GJ, Gribben JG, Gray G, Nadler LM (1993) Human T-cell clonal anergy is induced by antigen presentation in the absence of B7 costimulation. Proc Natl Acad Sci USA 90:6586–6590

Gückel B, Lindauer M, Rudy W, Habicht A, Siebels M, Kaul S, Bastert G, Meuer SC, Moebius U (1995) CD80-transfected human breast and ovarian tumor cell lines: improved immunogenicity and induction of cytolytic $CD8^+$ T lymphocytes. Cytokines Mol Ther 1:211–221

Habicht A, Lindauer M, Galmbacher P, Rudy W, Gebert J, Schackert H-K, Meuer SC, Moebius U (1995) Development of immunogenic colorectal cancer cell lines for vaccination: expression of CD80 (B7.1) is not sufficient to restore impaired primary T cell activation in vitro. Eur J Cancer 31A:2396–2402

Kawakami Y, Eliyahu S, Delgado CH, Robbins PF, Rivoltini L, Topalina SL, Miki T, Rosenberg SA (1994a) Cloning of the gene coding for a shared human melanoma antigen recognized by autologous T cell infiltrating into tumor. Proc Natl Acad Sci USA 91:3515–3519

Kawakami Y, Eliyahu S, Delgado CH, Robbins PF, Sakaguchi K, Appella E, Yanelli JR, Adema GJ, Miki T, Rosenberg SA (1994b) Identification of a human melanoma antigen recognized by tumor-infiltrating lymphocytes associated with in vivo tumor rejection. Proc Natl Acad Sci USA 91:6458–6462

Mueller DL, Jenkins MK, Schwartz RH (1989) Clonal expansion versus functional clonal inactivation; a costimulatory signalling pathway determines the outcome of T cell antigen receptor occupancy. Annu Rev Immunol 7:455–480

Pantel K, Schlimok G, Schaller G, Genz T, Wiebecke B, Backmann R, Funke I, Riethmüller G (1991) Frequent down-regulation of major histocompatibility class I antigen expression on individual micrometastatic carcinoma cells. Cancer Res 51:4712–4715

Schirren C, Völpel AH, Meuer SC (1992) Spontaneous responsiveness to cytokines by human T cell leukemias. Leukemia 6:574–581

Schwartz RH (1990) A culture model for T lymphocyte clonal anergy. Science 248:1349–1356

Smith MEF, Marsch SGE, Bodmer JG, Gelsthorpe K (1989) Loss of HLA-A, B, C allele products and lymphocyte function-associated antigen 3 in colorectal neoplasias. Proc Natl Acad Sci USA 86:5557–5561

Tepper RI, Pattengale PK, Leder P (1989) Murine interleukin-4 displays potent anti-tumor activity in vitro. Cell 57:503–512

Townsend SE, Allison JP (1993) Tumor rejection after direct costimulation of $CD8^{+}$ T cells by B7-transfected melanoma cells. Science 259:368–370

Traversari C, van der Bruggen P, Luescher IF, Lurquin C, Chomez P, Van Pel A, De Plaen E, Amar-Costesec A, Boon T (1992) A nonapeptide encoded by human gene MAGE-1 is recognized on HLA-A1 by cytolytic T lymphocytes directed against tumor antigen MZ2-E. J Exp Med 176:1453–1457

Van der Bruggen P, Traversari C, Chomez P, Lurquin C, De Plaen E, van den Eynde B, Knuth A, Boon T (1991) A gene encoding an antigen recognized by cytolytic T lymphocytes on a human melanoma. Science 254:1643–1647

Wölfel T, Hauer M, Schneider J, Serrano M, Wölfel C, Klehmann-Hieb E, De Plean E, Hankeln T, Meyer zum Büschenfelde K-H, Beach D (1995) A p16INK4a-insensitive CDK4 mutant targeted by cytolytic T lymphocytes in human melanoma. Science 269:1281–1284

Adeno-associated Virus Type 2 Vector for Transduction of Hematopoietic Cells

E. Ogniben[1] and R. Haas[1,2]

[1] Department of Internal Medicine V, University of Heidelberg, Hospitalstraße 3, 69115 Heidelberg, Germany
[2] German Cancer Research Center, Im Neuenheimer Feld 280, 69120 Heidelberg, Germany

Introduction

Recent advances in our understanding of the molecular basis of malignant diseases and the development of methods for constructing and transferring genes into mammalian cells has introduced the possibility of correcting genetic defects at the molecular level. Gene transfer into human pluripotent hematopoietic stem cells in particular represents a novel approach to gene therapy for some genetic or acquired diseases. To date, a major obstacle to stem-cell-targeted gene therapy in humans has been the low efficiency of transduction, especially in the quiescent stem cell population. The advantage of a viral vector is that it uses the natural ability of viruses to transfer their genetic material into cells after infection. Adeno-associated virus (AAV) vectors are promising candidates for the mediation of gene therapy of pluripotent hematopoietic stem cells, as they have been found capable of transducing nondividing cells (Podsakoff et al. 1994), especially nonproliferating respiratory epithelial cells (Flotte et al. 1994) and other cells such as postmitotic neurons (Du et al. 1996).

AAV is a single-stranded DNA virus with a genome size of 4680 nucleotides (Muzyczka 1992). Productive infection usually requires coinfection with adenovirus or herpesvirus, which provide helper functions for viral replication. An interesting aspect of the AAV life cycles is the fact that the viral DNA can integrate into the cellular genome during AAV infection in the absence of helper virus. Once integrated, the provirus is essentially quiescent until the cell is superinfected with adenovirus, whereupon the provirus is rescued. The following properties represent a basis for the development of AAV as a gene vector system for hematopoietic stem cells: so far, AAV has not been implicated as the causative agent of any known disease. AAV has a broad host range; in the absence of helper virus, the wild-type AAV genome integrates via the inverted terminal repeat into a unique region of the long arm of the human chromosome 19 (Samulski et al. 1991). A further advantage of recombinant AAV vectors (rAAVs) is their stable structure, they can be concentrated and purified.

Recent Results in Cancer Research, Vol. 144

Construction of the rAAV-*β-gal* Vector and Generation and Titration of rAAVs

For the purpose of using this system for gene therapy in patients with hematological malignancies, experiments with a reporter gene were performed. In an AAV vector, the entire protein-coding domain (±4.5 kb) can be replaced by the gene of interest, leaving only the flanking terminal repeats intact. We constructed a vector containing the *β*-galactosidase (*β-gal*) gene on the basis of the plasmid psub201 (Samulski et al. 1987) including a nuclear localization signal, under the control of the human cytomegalovirus promoter. The expression of the gene as well as another reporter gene, the green fluorescence protein, were first tested in transient transfection experiments. With a modified calcium-phosphate transfection method (Chen and Okayama 1987), transfection efficiencies between 50% and 60% could be achieved using the 293 line, an adenovirus-transformed human embryonic kidney cell line. The standard protocol for generation of recombinant AAV particles was used according to Rolling and Samulski (Rolling and Samulski 1995). For this, the recombinant plasmid encoding the *β-gal* is cotransfected with the helper plasmid called pAAV/Ad into 293 cells. The plasmid pAAV/Ad contains the *rep* and *cap* genes of the AAV genome as well as the adenovirus inverted terminal repeats, so that it cannot be packaged. The vector plasmid and the helper plasmid are cotransfected into adenoinfected tissue culture cells. In the presence of adenovirus, the rep proteins rescue and amplify the recombinant AAV genome from the vector plasmid, yielding a large pool of replicative-form DNA. The cap proteins sequester single-stranded rAAV genomes into a preformed virion, thus producing an infectious particle. After 48–72 h, cells show a cytopathic effect from adenoinfection and are harvested by low-speed centrifugation. Most of the rAAVs are cell-associated, and therefore the cell pellet is frozen and thawed three times, while the lysate is heated at 56 °C for 60 min to inactivate adenovirus. Since there is no homology between the helper plasmid and the AAV vector, we generated wild-type free recombinant AAV.

In order to determine the recombinant virus titers generated by the packaging procedure, a dot blot assay was used (Fig. 1). For that purpose, a permissive cell line like the cervical carcinoma cell line Hela was seeded in order to infect the cells with recombinant AAV particles in serial dilutions. After 2 h, the cells were superinfected with medium containing wild-type AAV and adenovirus, leading to amplification of the recombinant AAV genome. After lysing of the cells and DNA extraction, supernatant was blotted on a nylon membrane and hybridized with a specific radioactive-labeled lacZ probe. The blot was exposed and an autoradiograph was performed. The titers obtained were between 10^5 and 10^6 transducing particles per milliliter as assessed by Hela cell transduction on the basis of dot blot hybridization (Fig. 2). With a sulfonated cellulose column first described by Tamayose et al. (1996) it was possible to concentrate rAAVs up to 100-fold as shown in Fig. 3.

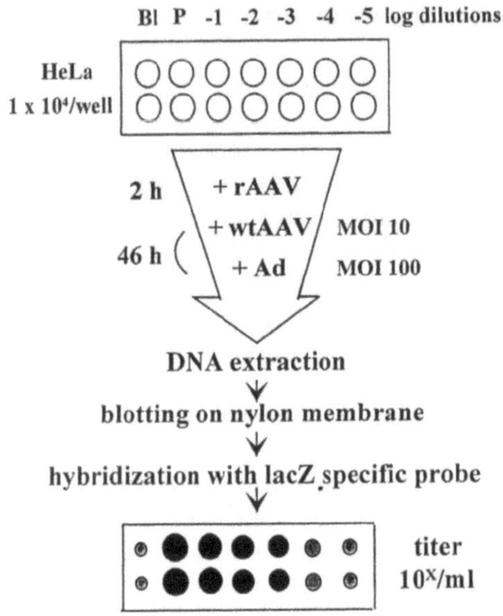

Fig. 1. Dot blot assay for titration of recombinant AAV particles

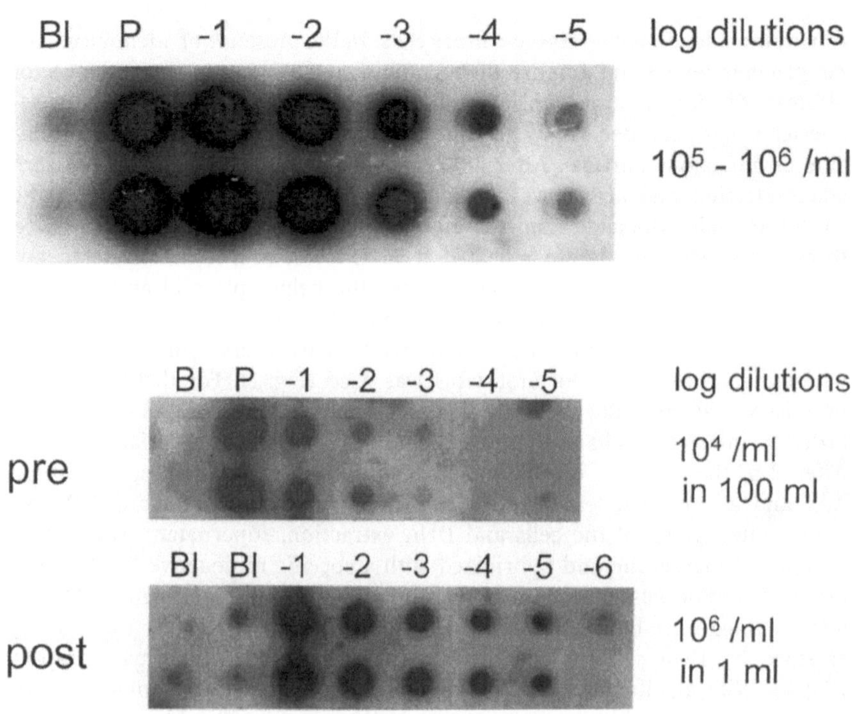

Fig. 3. Concentration of rAAV by sulfonated cellulose column

Transduction Experiments

With these lacZ particles, transduction experiments with the epithelial cell line Hela and a hematopoietic cell line K562 were performed. The adherent cervical carcinoma cell line Hela was transduced with an efficiency of about 30% (Fig. 4) without superinfection with adenovirus. When the cells were additionally infected with adenovirus, the transduction efficiency was approximately 80% (Fig. 5). In the mesenchymal cell line K562, as a model for transduction of hematopoietic cells, the transduction efficiency without adding adenovirus was about 5% (Fig. 6). In order to find an explanation for the lower transduction in mesenchymal cells, we performed immunofluorescence analysis with an anti-AAV capsid antibody after binding of wild-type AAV with a multiplicity of infection (MOI) of 100 in Hela cells and K562 cells. We found that Hela cells bound wild-type AAV in a greater proportion than K562 cells. Whether this finding relates to greater expression of an as yet uncloned AAV receptor on epithelial cells in comparison to mesenchymal cells is not known.

Conclusions

Recently, Fisher et al. (1996) showed that adenovirus significantly enhanced rAAV transduction in vitro dependent on expression of early region 1 and 4 (E1 and E4, respectively) genes and in direct proportion to the appearance of double-stranded replicative forms of the rAAV genome. Another group

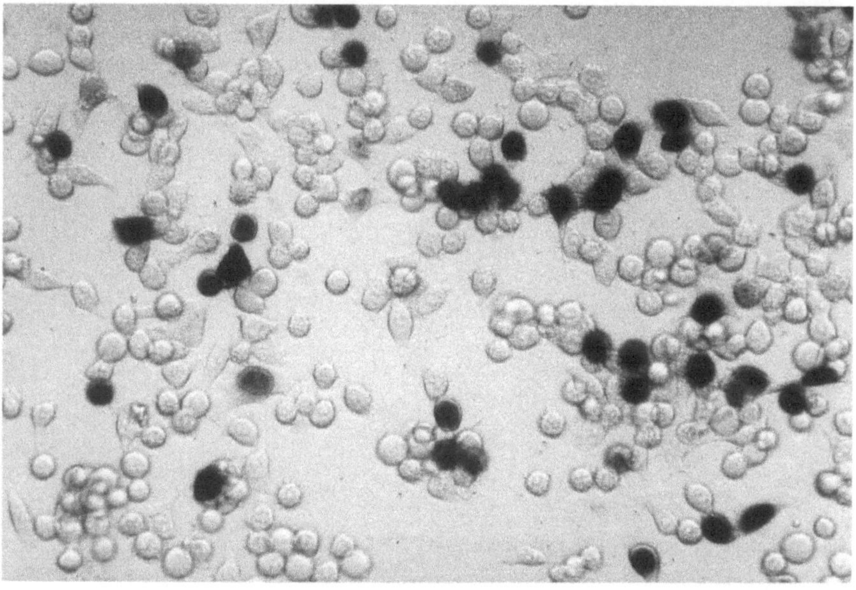

Fig. 4. Transduction with rAAV lacZ cervix carcinoma cell line Hela (MOI 1)

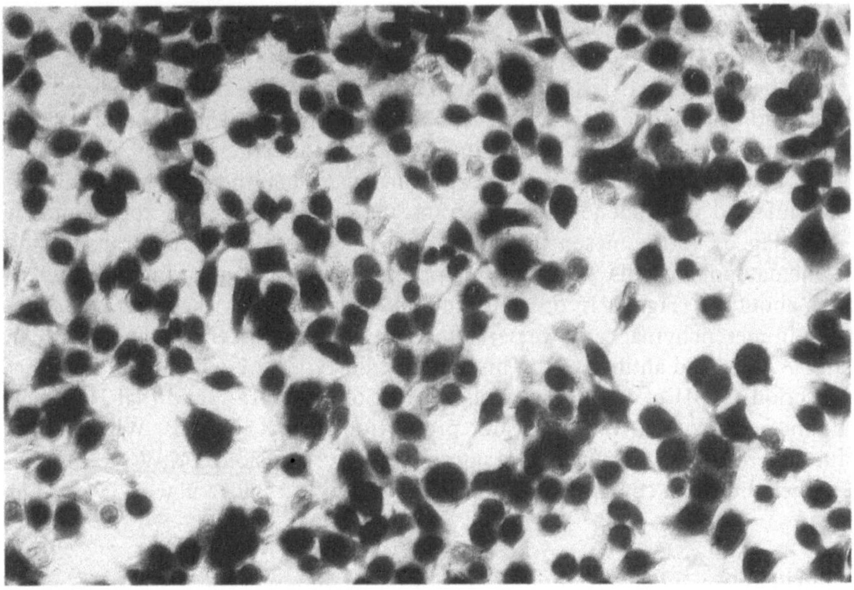

Fig. 5. Transduction with rAAV lacZ cervix carcinoma cell line Hela (multiplicity of infection, MOI 1) with superinfection using adenovirus

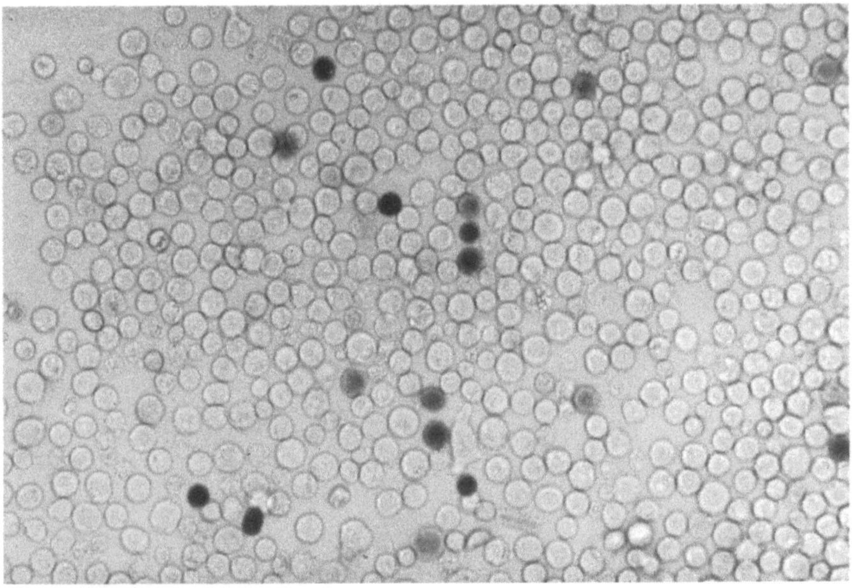

Fig. 6. Transduction with rAAV lacZ erythroleukemia cell line K562 (MOI 1)

showed an approximately 1000-fold increase in transduction frequency when cells were co-infected with adenovirus or exposed to genotoxic or/and physical stress (Ferrari et al. 1996). Halbert et al. (1995) showed that AAV vectors transduced primary cells much less efficiently than immortalized cells. Indeed, for transduction of primary hematopoietic cells, efficient transduction requires greater multiplicity of infection to ensure excess of biologically active vector particles over the target cell population. Efforts are currently geared towards the generation of recombinant AAV particles with higher titers by using concentrating and purification steps like caesium chloride gradients. Other groups tried to generate packaging cell lines containing the gene of interest and the *rep* and *cap* genes or the use of adenovirus linked to the helper plasmid. But even with these packaging cell lines it was not possible to produce recombinant AAVs with higher titers. Assessment of new helper plasmids which enhance the expression of the AAV genes is under way.

First transduction experiments with CD34+ cells from patients having undergone cytotoxic chemotherapy with G-CSF support have been performed. Due to the low MOI only a few transduced cells were occasionally observed after 48 h coincubation of the cells with rAAVs. Whether stimulation of the target cells with cytokines is necessary for efficient transduction has not been answered yet. Russell et al. (1994) showed that AAV vectors preferentially transduced cells in S-phase, whereas other groups found no relationship between transduction and the proliferation status of the cell (Podsakoff et al. 1994). To enhance transduction in primary nondividing cells, some authors used DNA-damaging agents to induce DNA repair mechanisms (Alexander et al. 1994; Russell et al. 1995).

Successful transduction of CD34+ cells has been reported by different groups. Miller et al. (1994) found transgene expression in 20%–40% of hematopoietic colonies following transduction with a recombinant AAV vector encoding human γ-globin. Walsh et al. (1994) observed a transduction efficiency of 60%. Recently, it was shown that AAV vectors integrate in CD34+ human hematopoietic progenitor cells after transduction (Fisher-Adams et al. 1996). It will be important to use standardized purified AAV vectors to determine better conditions for efficient and safe transduction of CD34+ cells, thus to provide a basis for ex vivo gene therapy of the hematopoietic system.

Acknowledgment. We are indebted to Jürgen Kleinschmidt and his coworkers for their assistance with vector construction and for fruitful discussions.

References

Alexander IE, Russel DW, Miller AD (1994) DNA-damaging agents greatly increased the transduction of nondividing cells by adeno-associated virus vectors. J Virol 68:8282–8287

Chen D, Okayama H (1987) High-efficiency transformation of mammalian cells by plasmid DNA. Mol Cell Biol 7:2745–2752

Du B, Wu P, Boldt-Houle DM, Terwilliger EF (1996) Efficient transduction of human neurons with an adeno-associated virus vector. Gene Ther 3:254–261

Ferrari FK, Samulski T, Shenk T, Samulski RJ (1996) Second-strand synthesis is a rate-limiting step for efficient transduction by recombinant adeno-associated virus vectors. J Virol 70:3227–3234

Fisher KJ, Gao GP, Weitzman MD, DeMatteo R, Burda JF, Wilson JM (1996) Transduction with recombinant adeno-associated virus for gene therapy is limited by leading-strand synthesis. J Virol 70:520–532

Fisher-Adams G, Wong KK Jr, Podsakoff G, Forman SJ, Chatterjee S (1996) Integration of adeno-associated virus vectors in CD34+ human hematopoietic progenitor cells after transduction. Blood 88:492–504

Flotte TR, Afione SA, Zeitlin PL (1994) Adeno-associated virus vector gene expression occurs in nondividing cells in the absence of vector DNA integration. Am J Respir Cell Mol Biol 11:517–521

Halbert CL, Alexander IE, Wolgamot GM, Miller AD (1995) Adeno-associated virus vectors transduce primary cells much less efficiently than immortalized cells. J Virol 69:1473–1479

Miller JL, Donahue RE, Sellers SE, Samulski RJ, Young NS, Nienhuis AW (1994) Recombinant adeno-associated virus (rAAV)-mediated expression of a human γ-globin gene in human progenitor-derived erythroid cells. Proc Natl Acad Sci USA 91:10183–10187

Muzyczka N (1992) Use of adeno-associated virus as a general transduction vector for mammalian cells. Curr Top Microbiol Immunol 158:97–129

Podsakoff G, Wong KK Jr, Chatterjee S (1994) Efficient gene transfer into nondividing cells by adeno-associated virus-based vectors. J Virol 68:5656–5666

Rolling F, Samulski RJ (1995) AAV as a viral vector for human gene therapy. Mol Biotechnol 3:9–15

Russell DW, Miller AD, Alexander IE (1994) Adeno-associated virus vectors preferentially transduce cells in S-phase. Proc Natl Acad Sci USA 91:8915–8919

Russell DW, Alexander IE, Miller AD (1995) DNA synthesis and topoisomerase inhibitors increase transduction by adeno-associated virus vector. Proc Natl Acad Sci USA 92:5719–5723

Samulski RJ, Chang LS, Shenk T (1987) A recombinant plasmid from which an infectious adeno-associated virus genome can be excised in vitro and its use to study viral replication. J Virol 61:3096–3101

Samulski RJ, Zhu X, Xiao X, Brook JD, Housman DE, Epstein N, Hunter LA (1991) Targeted integration of adeno-associated virus (AAV) into human chromosome 19. EMBO J 10:3941–3950

Tamayose K, Hirai Y, Shimada T (1996) A new strategy for large-scale preparation of high-titer recombinant adeno-associated virus vectors by using packaging cells lines and sulfonated cellulose column chromatography. Hum Gene Ther 7:507–513

Walsh CE, Nienhuis AW, Samulski RJ, Brown MG, Miller JL (1994) Phenotypic correction of Fanconi anemia in human hematopoietic cells with a recombinant adeno-associated virus vector. J Clin Invest 94:1440–1448

Protection of Hematopoietic Stem Cells from Chemotherapy-Induced Toxicity by Multidrug-Resistance 1 Gene Transfer

S. Fruehauf[1], K. Wermann[2], E.C. Buss[2], P. Hundsdoerfer[2], M.R. Veldwijk[2], R. Haas[1], and W.J. Zeller[2]

[1] Department of Internal Medicine V, University of Heidelberg, Hospitalstraße 3, 69115 Heidelberg, Germany
[2] German Cancer Research Center, Department 0420, Im Neuenheimer Feld 280, Heidelberg, Germany

Abstract

An increased chemotherapeutic dose intensity is believed to translate into higher survival rates among cancer patients. Pancytopenia is the dose-limiting toxic result of most anticancer agents. Overexpression of the human multidrug resistance 1 (*MDR*1) gene in transgenic animals resulted in complete myeloprotection against high doses of cytostatic drugs. Stem cell research, vector development, and experimental pharmacology are uniting their efforts in an attempt to achieve a similar effect in human hematopoietic stem cells. This article gives an overview of the crucial steps involved, from retroviral vector design and optimization of viral titers to vector uptake, gene integration, and expression. The authors' own results are presented with special regard in vitro and in vivo assays for the detection of hematopoietic stem cell transduction.

The Concept of "Protective" Gene Transfer

Drug resistance genes were first recognized because their expression created major obstacles to the successful treatment of cancer. Initially, research focused on the inhibition of gene function in malignant cells, with the aim of increasing their sensitivity to chemotherapy relative to that of normal tissues, i.e., to increase the therapeutic index. However, tissues that are naturally protected by detoxifying mechanisms, such as hematopoietic stem cells, may also be affected by the systemic application of sensitizing agents and become more vulnerable to the ensuing chemotherapy, with resultant prolonged cytopenia. This dilemma was the starting point from which alternatives were sought.

One idea was to protect normal cells by transferring drug-resistance genes into the cells (Fig. 1). The proof-of-principle experiment was performed by the group of Gottesman and Pastan at the National Institutes of Health in Bethesda (Galski et al. 1989). They chose for the multidrug resistance gene

Recent Results in Cancer Research, Vol. 144

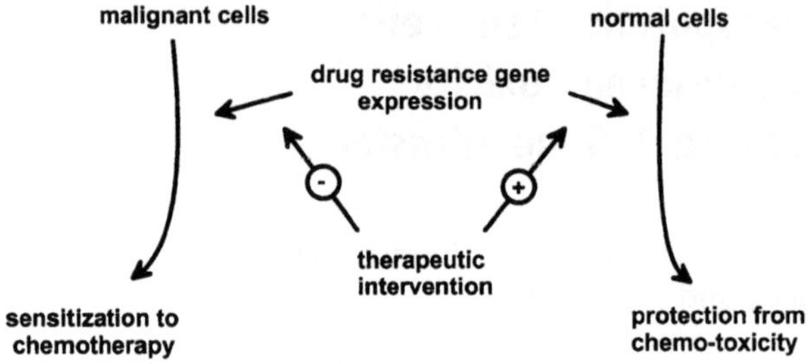

Fig. 1. Modulation of drug resistance gene expression in malignant or normal cells to increase the therapeutic index

*MDR*1, which encodes a 170-kDA membrane protein termed P-glycoprotein (Pgp). The protein acts as a transmembrane efflux pump, thus reducing the intracellular concentration of the drug. Pgp confers resistance to a wide array of lipophilic, yet structurally unrelated drugs such as taxanes, vinca alkaloids, and topoisomerase inhibitors. In a transgenic mouse model of P-glycoprotein overexpression, Galski et al. (1989) were able to show complete protection of the hematopoietic system to 8.5 mg daunorubicin per kilogram body weight, whereas the white blood cell count of normal control mice dropped to 35% of starting values on day 8.

The transfer of these encouraging findings to the patient situation required some modifications. Hematopoietic stem cells had to become the target of gene transfer instead of the germ line. This was rendered possible by seminal advances in stem cell research over the last decade. In 1984 Curt Civin and coworkers first described an antibody to KG1 leukemia cells. The recognized antigen was later termed CD34. CD34+ cells were demonstrated to mediate hematopoietic reconstitution following myeloablative therapy in humans (Berenson et al. 1991; Haas et al. 1994). Immunological methods were developed to physically separate CD34+ cells from bone marrow, peripheral blood, or leukapheresis products (Berenson et al. 1988; Civin et al. 1990; Fruehauf et al. 1994; Hohaus et al., this volume). Stepwise evolution and the clinical introduction of CD34+ cell selection and cytokine-mediated progenitor cell expansion have formed the basis for gene transfer studies to human hematopoietic stem cells.

At the same time, suitable shuttle systems for gene transfer had to be developed. Physical methods such as calcium phosphate precipitation, electroporation, or lipofection were not sufficiently effective. Replication-deficient retroviruses in which structural genes had been replaced by an inserted gene of interest and which were still able to infect hematopoietic stem cells efficiently through a specific receptor appeared the most promising. After extensive preclinical studies (van Beusechem et al. 1992) the group of Dinko Valerio in Leiden was the first to transplant gene-modified bone marrow cells into immunodeficient patients in 1992 (Hoogerbrugge et al. 1992). To date, close to half of the approved gene therapy trials involve gene transfer and transgene expression in hematopoietic cells. Gene-marking studies attempt to analyze the fate of cells delivered during transplantation of hematopoietic progenitors. The contribution of tumor cells in the graft to relapse following high-dose therapy was demonstrated for acute and chronic myeloid leukemia as well as neuroblastoma (Brenner et al. 1993; Deisseroth et al. 1994), which in turn stimulated the interest in tumor cell purging studies. Mobilized peripheral blood was demonstrated to contain more hematopoietic stem cells with long-term reconstitution potential than bone marrow (Dunbar et al. 1995). These studies focused on the detection of transferred genes in the progeny of the marked cells. However, it should be kept in mind that a gene-marking protocol cannot benefit the patient directly while it imposes potential hazards on the individual, such as the risk of insertional mutagenesis or malignant transformation (Donahue et al. 1992).

For the next step therapeutic genes that need to be expressed if possible at high levels were chosen. Now the worlds of high-dose chemotherapy and stem cell transplantation, vector technology, and knowledge about drug resistance genes could meet.

Several drug resistance genes have been cloned into viral vectors with the aim of chemotherapeutic dose-intensification and selection of transduced cells in vivo (Sorrentino et al. 1992). The multidrug resistance gene (*MDR*1) is a prime candidate for clinical application. So far, the wild-type *MDR*1 gene and a mutant *MDR*1 gene containing a point mutation resulting in a substitution of valine for glycine at codon 185 (Hanania et al. 1995; Ward et al. 1994) have been employed. The mutation results in decreased resistance to taxol and increased resistance to colchicine. Recently, a cryptic splice donor and splice acceptor site were identified in both the wild-type and the mutated *MDR*1 mRNA (Sorrentino et al. 1995). These cryptic splice sites were activated at very low frequency with transcription of genomic *MDR*1 sequences. In vector-derived transcripts up to 60% of the total vector-derived message was truncated. However, the full length *MDR*1 mRNA exceeded those from endogenous genes and were equivalent to that seen in the modestly drug-resistant cell line SW320 (Sorrentino et al. 1995). Of note for clinical application, the substrate specificity of its gene product P-glycoprotein varies substantially, e.g., a retrovirally *MDR*1-transduced cell line was resistant to a 290-fold higher concentration of taxol than untransduced control cells, while the resistance factor for vincristine was 100 and for etoposide 6.7 (Boesen et al. 1995).

Mutant forms of the dihydrofolate reductase (*DHFR*) gene confer resistance to methotrexate, an antifolate. It was observed that the mutant Ser31 *DHFR* cDNA (wild-type Phe31) was able to protect mice from methotrexate toxicity, and both secondary and tertiary recipients were also protected, indicating that this protection was due to transduction of an early progenitor or stem cell (Li et al. 1994). Following coculture of CD34+ peripheral blood cells on a Ser31 *DHFR* retroviral producer cell line and subsequent selection in methotrexate, the transduced cells showed a relative resistance factor of 4 compared to mock-transduced controls (Flasshove et al. 1995).

The aldehyde dehydrogenase-1 gene (*ALDH*1) detoxifies cyclophosphamide and its analog maphosphamide. Retroviral transfer of the *ALDH*1 gene into murine L1210 or human K562 leukemic cells allowed survival of these cells at concentrations of 5–25 μM maphosphamide in two studies (Magni et al. 1996; Web and Sorrentino 1994). In this context it is of note that for bone marrow purging in acute myelogenous leukemia concentrations of 80–100 μM maphosphamide are employed, which still results in survival of approximately 5% of the initial colony-forming progenitors.

A myeloproliferative sarcoma virus-based vector was used to express human O^6-alkylguanine DNA alkyltransferase (*MGMT*) cDNA in human or murine hematopoietic cells. *MGMT* is a nuclear protein, demethylating O^6-methylguanine formed after nitrosourea treatment of DNA (Samson 1992). The transfer of the alkyl group to the protein's essential SH group irreversibly inactivates the protein. After bone marrow transplant a persistent 10- to 40-fold increase of *MGMT* expression was observed, accompanied with an approximately 2-fold increased resistance of murine hematopoietic cells to BCNU treatment (Allay et al. 1995).

Transfection or transduction of a glutathione-S-transferase (*GST*) gene into NIH/3T3 fibroblasts conferred, respectively, 5.8- and 2.4-fold resistance to chlorambucil and 10.8- and 5.4-fold resistance to mechlorethamine (Greenbaum et al. 1994).

Further nononcological indications for gene therapy include inherited disorders of hematopoietic cells such as hemoglobinopathies, immune deficiency syndromes, lysosomal storage disorders, mucopolysaccharidoses, and acquired immune deficiency disorders.

All these concepts are quite elaborate. However, the technology to meet the goals is still in an early developmental phase. This article gives an overview on issues in vector design and stem cell transduction that have to be considered for efficient "protective" gene transfer.

The Gene Transfer System

Retroviral Vectors

Retroviral vectors currently represent the most widely applied and – as regards biological safety and efficacy – best characterized system for somatic gene transfer (see Günzburg et al., this volume). At present, vectors are most frequently derived from Moloney murine leukemia virus (MoMLV), a mouse type C retrovirus (Baum and Ostertag 1996).

Vector Design

The retroviral genome harbors at least three structural genes, *gag, pol,* and *env.* These genes are flanked by two direct long terminal repeats (LTRs) that, besides other functions, contain promoter/enhancer elements for transcription. All three genes can be deleted and replaced by a transgene, e.g., a therapeutic gene (see Fig. 2). Only the LTRs and the packaging signal remain in the vector; they are termed "cis-acting elements." Vectors can accommodate inserted transgenes of up to 9 kb in size. The cis-acting elements required for packaging and reverse transcription comprise approximately 1 kb. Following integration the stability and gene expression from the provirus is determined by these sequences. Enhancer/promotor elements can be placed in the U3-region of the LTR or in the transgene. If the enhanced/promotor is located in the U3-region of the LTR, 3′ flanking genes can be activated and insertional mutagenesis could result. If internal promotors are used the U3 region can be deleted, which results in nonmobilizable vectors, because genomic RNA cannot be formed following transduction. However, due to low virus titers, these otherwise attractive self-inactivating vectors have received limited attention (Faustinella et al. 1994; Russ et al. 1996).

Single-gene vectors are the most common type of vector. They are useful only if the therapeutic gene can function by itself as selection marker, which is the case for, e.g., the *MDR*1 gene. Baum et al. (1995) determined the expression of a *MDR*1 gene cloned into different novel retroviral expression constructs. Expression was controlled by either Friend mink cell focus-forming virus or myeloproliferative sarcoma virus enhancer sequences combined with the primer binding site of murine embryonic stem cell virus. In hematopoietic cell lines the hybrid vectors provided about a three-fold higher protection against the *MDR*1-related drug colchicine compared to MoMLV-derived regulatory sequences (Eckert et al. 1996).

Double-gene vectors harbor two genes, a selectable marker and the therapeutic gene. Either both genes can be driven the retroviral LTRs or each gene can be driven by its own promoter element. Practically, this approach does not allow efficient control of gene expression (Emerman and Temin 1986). Bicistronic vectors allow the expression of two cistrons from one mRNA. The downstream cistron is preceded by an internal ribosomal entry site of, e.g., encephalomyocarditis virus (Dirks et al. 1993; Koo et al. 1992; Levine et al. 1991; Metz et al. 1996; Morgan et al. 1992; Sugimoto et al. 1994; Torrent et al. 1996). Other expression strategies for double-gene vectors include alternative splicing or LTR minigenes. For general reviews on vector systems, the reader is referred to Uckert and Walther (1994), Valerio (1992), or Jolly (1994). Approaches for targeting to other organs (e.g., to liver or mammary gland) have recently been reviewed (Miller and Vile 1995; Salmons et al. 1995; Salmons and Günzburg 1993).

Retroviral Packaging Systems

The trans-acting viral structure proteins responsible for packaging, target cell interaction, uptake, nuclear translocation, and eventually integration of the vector genome are provided by packaging cell lines. The resulting vectors are replication-incompetent, because the genetic information for the trans-acting proteins is not conferred (Fig. 2).

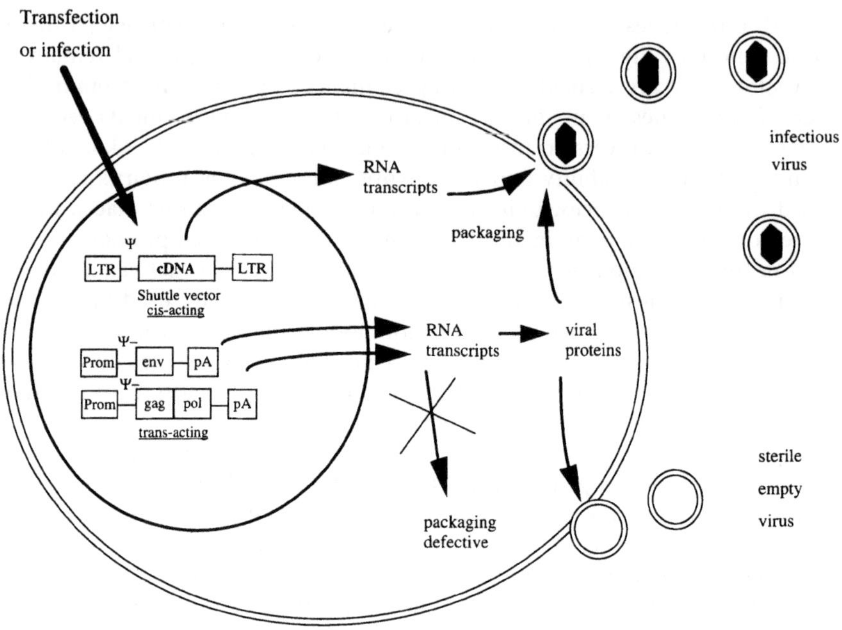

Fig. 2. Retroviral packaging cell line: cis and trans acting elements (adapted from Valerio 1992). A packaging cell at work. A retroviral vector carrying all of the in cis requirements as well as the gene(s) of interest is introduced into the packaging cell. This can be achieved either by physical transfection or by infection with a recombinant retrovirus whose entrance is not hindered by interference. The packaging cell produces all of the viral proteins itself, but generates no functional virus particles. Transcripts from the vector, however, can be packaged by the virus proteins to form infectious virus. Virus stocks from such cells are therefore helper-free and the recombinant retroviruses are replication-defective, so they can only undergo the first stages of the viral life cycle

MoMLV based retroviral vectors carry some critical features that need to be regarded for successful gene transfer. First, they can only infect dividing cells, a feature that might be useful for targeting fast-growing cancer cells but a hurdle for gene therapy of quiescent hematopoietic stem cells. Secondly, viral particles are unstable, disintegrating at 37 °C within a few hours, and hence cannot be concentrated efficiently by, e.g., ultracentrifugation. Third, viral particles derived from murine 3T3 cells are inactivated by the complement of human serum, precluding in vivo delivery. The most important point to consider is the generation of contaminating replication-competent retroviral particles (RCR). RCR can be released from packaging cell lines after recombinational events between helper virus DNA sequences and vector DNA, which is added by the presence of endogenous retroviral sequences in the genome of murine 3T3 cells, which most packaging cell lines are derived from. The possibility of successful recombination can be minimized by physically separating retroviral *gag-pol* genes from *env* genes within the host genome, so that two or more recombinations are required to produce RCR. For this reason, redundant genetic material should be deleted from the retroviral sequences.

The host range of retroviruses is determined by the binding specificities of the retroviral envelope protein (the product of the *env*-gene). The SU subunit of the envelope protein establishes the target cell contact while the TM subunit is responsible for uptake into the cytoplasm. The envelope protein recognizes a phosphate transporter which is expressed in a differentiation-dependent fashion on the target cells.

Ecotropic viruses infect mouse cells and - to a lesser extent - rat cells. Amphotropic viruses have a wider host range, including mouse, monkey, and man. Xenotropic viruses, derived from mouse cells, have a wide host range, including monkey and man, but do not infect mouse cells. For a review on retroviral receptors and envelope proteins see Weiss and Tailor (1995) and references cited therein.

Three widely used packaging cell lines are PA317, GP+envAM12, and PG13, all of which were generated from mouse 3T3 fibroblasts. The amphotropic line PA317 (Miller and Buttimore 1986) harbors a single helper genome from which the packaging signal and the 3′-LTR was deleted. Generation of RCR has been observed on rare occasions with this line. According to Xu et al. (1994) retroviral supernatants derived from the PA317 inhibit growth of bone marrow CD34+ cells, therapy reducing transduction efficiency five-fold compared with supernatants derived from line GP+envAM12 of the same viral titers. This effect was ameliorated when anti-transforming growth factor-β antibodies were included in the PA317-derived supernatant.

The amphotropic line GP+envAM12 and the ecotropic line GP+E86 (Markowitz et al. 1988a,b), harbor two separate proviral DNA constructs supplying either *gag-pol* or *env* functions, and the amphotropic line Psi-CRIP and the ecotropic line Psi-CRE (Danos and Mulligan 1988) harbor two proviral DNA constructs carrying complementary mutations in *gag-pol* and *env* sequences. Both ecotropic lines are frequently used to transduce their amphotropic counterparts. However, the risk of RCR formation increases with every ping-pong infection.

For construction of the line PG13 (Miller et al. 1991), MoMLV *gag-pol* sequences as well as gibbon ape leukemia virus (GALV) *env* sequences were sequentially introduced into 3T3 cells. Because the host range of the recombinant viral particles includes human cells, but does not include 3T3 mouse cells, the risk of possible RCR spreading in the packaging cell cultures is reduced. Line PG13 was reported to be superior to line PA317 for the transduction of human bone marrow cells, which may be due to a higher expression of the GALV receptor (Glvr-1) than the amphotropic receptor (Ram-1) (Kozak et al. 1995; Miller and Miller 1994; von Kalle et al. 1994). Miller and Chen (1996) described a new packaging cell line in which the *gag-pol* genes of MoMLV are combined with the *env* gene of the 10A1 strain of MLV, which promotes entrance via two receptors, the amphotropic receptor and GALV receptor, possibly resulting in higher gene transfer efficiencies.

One further approach to improve virus-cell interactions are targeted molecular genetic alterations in the SU domain of the env protein (Cosset et al. 1995; Russel 1996).

How to Optimize Viral Titers

Retroviral vectors are obtained as cell-free supernatant from packaging cells. For determination of viral titers, a permissive cell line (often NIH/3T3) is infected using serial dilutions of retroviral supernatant. Thereafter the number of marker-resistant colonies is determined. Titers are given as drug-resistant colony-forming units per milliliter of viral stock (Fig. 3). Alternatively, fluorescent dyes such as rhodamine-123 may be employed, which are transported out of the cell via the P-glycoprotein pump (Fig. 4).

The optimum cellular density during harvest of retroviral supernatant, the amount and type of medium, and the time for vector production are crucial. Floating cells and cellular debris should be minimal as they release proteases and RNAses that lead to the disintegration of retroviral vectors. Retroviral particles are unstable in cell culture media. Therefore, harvesting virus particles at 32 °C instead of 37 °C may improve stability, and hence up to ten-fold higher viral titers can be expected despite a reduced release of viral particles from the packaging cells (Kotani et al. 1994). The medium composition also appears to influence the vector production and needs to be optimized for individual applications (Fig. 5).

To eliminate microbial contaminants, retroviral supernatants should be sterilized by filtration through 0.45-μm-pore-size filters and kept at 0 °C before application. Although the use of fresh retroviral supernatants is recommended, shock-freezing and storage at –70 °C in liquid nitrogen or lyophilization (Kotani et al. 1994) are possible.

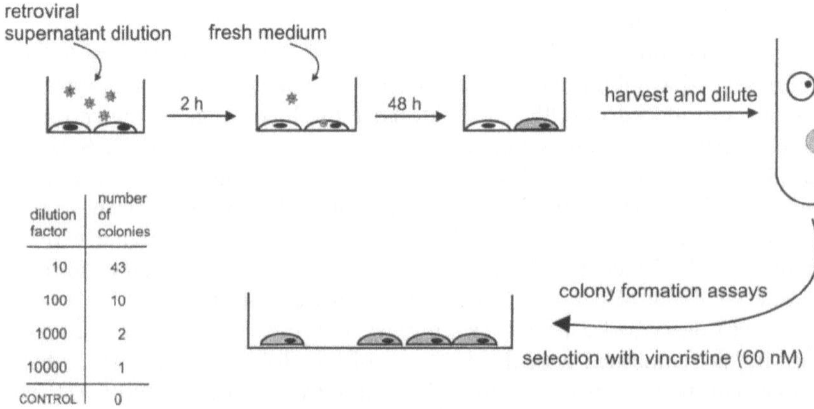

Fig. 3. Retroviral vectors are obtained as cell-free supernatant from packaging cells. For determination of viral titers, a permissive cell line (often NIH/3T3) is infected using serial dilutions of retroviral supernatant. Thereafter the number of marker-resistant colonies is determined. Titers are given as drug-resistant colony-forming units per milliliter of viral stock. e.g., 10^4 viral particles per milliliter in this example

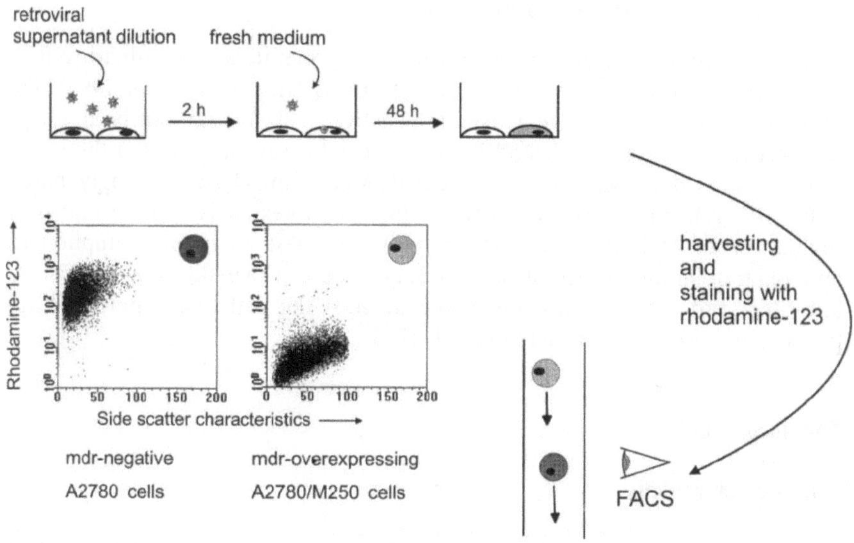

Fig. 4. Following transduction with a retroviral *MDR*1 supernatant, cells can be stained with the fluorescent dye rhodamine-123. Transduced cells are able to extrude the dye and become rhodamine-123^{dull}, while untransduced cells retain the dye in their cytoplasm

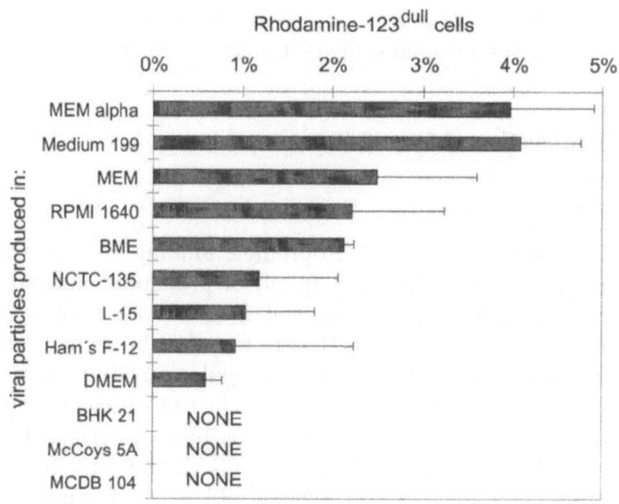

Fig. 5. Optimization of retroviral *MDR*1 supernatant harvesting includes testing of different tissue culture media

How to Screen for Replication-Competent Retroviruses

Using appropriate cell and molecular biological methods contaminating RCR can be detected at a sensitivity of 10^{-7} particles (Anderson et al. 1993). For example, a sarcoma-positive, leukemia-negative (S+L–) assay can be used. By coculture of packaging cells and indicator cells for several passages the sensitivity of RCR detection can be increased. Most clinical studies apply maximally 10^9 transducing vector particles. In this context it is of note that only high titers of MoMLV-related RCRs (10^7) were able to induce lymphomas, and only in immune-incompetent primate hosts (Cornetta et al. 1993). At low titers and with an immune-competent host the pathogenic potential appears to be negligible (Anderson et al. 1993).

The Target Cell

Source of Stem Cells

Stem cells can be obtained from normal bone marrow before the onset of chemotherapy, or from bone marrow or peripheral blood in the recovery phase after chemotherapy and/or cytokine stimulation (G-CSF, GM-CSF, or SCF/G-CSF) (Dunbar et al. 1996; Lu et al. 1994; Nolta et al. 1995; Hohaus et al., this volume). Furthermore, umbilical cord blood is a source of primitive stem cells that receives considerable interest for gene therapy (Hanley et al. 1994; Shi et al. 1994). To increase the vector-to-target cell ratio most groups use CD 34+-selected cells for transduction studies.

Transduction of Stem Cells

Retrovirus Vectors

Vector Binding and Uptake. To promote binding of viral particles to their cellular receptors, polybrene (1–8 µg/ml) or protamine sulfate (4–8 µg/ml) are added. In some studies protamine sulfate (Flasshove et al. 1995) as well as cationic lipids (Dybing et al. 1995) were found to be superior to polybrene. A 30/35-kDa fragment of fibronectin (a cellular matrix protein) used for coating the plates was shown to improve transduction efficiency, possibly by enabling co-localization of stem cells and virus particles (Hanenberg et al. 1996; Moritz et al. 1994, 1996). Viral supernatants can be centrifuged onto a monolayer of target cells for 1–4 h at 1000×g and 32 °C (Bunnell et al. 1995; Chuck and Palsson 1996; Kotani et al. 1994) or – at least in some cases – be concentrated as described (Paul et al. 1993; see also van Beusechem et al. 1993). Since binding of retroviruses to the cellular receptor is limited by retroviral stability and diffusion rate in the static culture vessels, binding can be increased using a net fluid flow of retrovirus-containing medium through a layer of target cells (Palsson et al. 1995).

Despite high viral titers, transduction efficiencies of target cells can be low, possibly due to low amounts of viral receptor proteins on the cellular surface. Especially the amphotropic receptor Ram-1 seems to be expressed poorly on phenotypically primitive CD34+/CD38– cells (Orlic et al. 1996). Its expression can be upregulated by incubation of target cells in phosphate-free medium for 1–2 days and, in cells lacking the receptor, can be transiently achieved by using an receptor-transducing adenoviral vector (Lieber et al. 1995). However, the use of the latter approach for human hematopoietic cells is questionable, since infectious adenoviral particles can appear (Mitani et al. 1994). Cytokines were also able to upregulate the amphotropic retrovirus receptor on hematopoietic cells, with IL-3 being the most important one (Crooks and Kohn 1993).

Vector Integration. Following uptake via a specific receptor, retroviral genomic RNA is transcribed to double-stranded DNA in the cytoplasm. The nuclear translocation of the preintegration complex requires the breakdown of the nuclear membrane and mitosis of the target cells. Hematopoietic stem cells are mostly in the quiescent phase of the cell cycle and require cytokines for proliferation induction.

In study by our group mobilized peripheral blood progenitor cells were primarily found to be in the resting phase of the cell cycle (Fruehauf et al. 1996). Incubation in the presence of hematopoietic growth factors induced cell cycle progression of CD34+ cells from below 5% in the S/G_2M-phase to above 30% after 48 h. As expected, integration of the transgene *MDR*1 and cell cycle activation were in correlation. We did not observe a difference in cell cycle activation following incubation in interleukin-3 (IL-3, 50 ng/ml), stem cell factor (SCF, 100 ng/ml)+IL-3 (50 ng/ml), or SCF (100 ng/ml)+IL-6 (50 ng/ml)+IL-3 (20 ng/ml). Others used various cytokines in a wide concentration range – e.g., IL-3 (5–100 ng/ml), IL-6 (50–200 ng/ml), SCF (50–100 ng/ml), IL-1 (50–100 ng/ml) – with comparable results in many studies, pointing to other common limiting factors for vector integration, such as low retrovirus receptor expression or viral titers.

Since the highest rate of proliferation induction occurs within the first 48 h, with a less pronounced further increase to 96 h, most groups use these time intervals for transduction of blood or marrow progenitors (e.g., Dunbar et al. 1996; Hanania et al. 1995; Hanley et al. 1994; Hughes et al. 1992; Moritz et al. 1994; Nolta et al. 1995; Shi et al. 1994; Ward et al. 1994; Xu et al. 1995). Due to the short vector half-life at 37 °C, fresh supernatant needs to be added every 12–24 h. The addition of bone marrow stroma or stromal factors during transduction appears advantageous as they may prevent terminal differentiation and thus preserve the repopulation potential of the graft (Moore et al. 1992; Nolta et al. 1995; Xu et al. 1995). Stromal factors may even be required for the transduction of some primitive stem cell subsets in bone marrow (Nolta et al. 1995). An alternative to primary bone marrow stroma cells are human unbilical vein endothelial cells (Sekhar et al. 1995) or bone-marrow-derived stroma cell lines (Bertolini et al. 1996; Kodama et al. 1984; Pulsipher et al. 1995; van Germeraad et al. 1994).

A long-term culture (1–3 weeks) can increase transduction efficiencies, as it allows more stem cells to enter S-phase. For this approach, long-term bone marrow cultures (LTBMC) were established from bone marrow low-density mononuclear cells. Fresh retroviral supernatant of packaging line PG13/LN was fed once a day for up to 3 weeks and IL-1, IL-3, IL-6, SCF (each at 50 ng/ml), and polybrene (4 μg/ml) were added. High transduction efficiencies (63%–100%) of long-term culture-initiating cells were reported using this approach (von Kalle et al. 1994). In a murine system, efficient repopulation of bone marrow of lethally irradiated B6 mice was reported using LTBMC in a transwell coculture system at 33 °C plus GP+E86/W5 packaging cells, followed by G418 selection for a total of 15–18 days in ex vivo culture (van Germeraad et al. 1994). Kiem et al. (1994) reported the repopulation of bone marrow of two out of three dogs with stem cells after transduction with PA317/LN in an LTBMC system (Schuening et al. 1989). Peripheral blood progenitor cells were mobilized with SCF and transduced for 11 days with fresh retroviral supernatant given every other day, followed by intravenous infusion of cells at day 11.

Another approach to achieving nuclear translocation of retroviral vectors in noncycling cells is to use properties of HIV and related lentiviruses (Lewis et al. 1992; Naldini et al. 1996). The HIV matrix-gag protein provides a translocation signal which is considered to allow active transportation across nuclear pores. This does not, however, seem to be sufficient for the infection of quiescent cells, as metabolically active macrophages and neurons were found to be HIV-infected, but not resting T cells or stem cells. Further research in this field is directed towards the use of non-human-pathogenic lenti- and spumaviruses.

Expression of the Provirus. The expression of a transferred gene can be studied with in vitro assays for human hematopoietic stem cells or with human-mouse transplantation chimaerae (Fig. 6). The colony-forming ability is a marker of the short-term reconstitution potential of an autograft. Cells are grown in semisolid media over 14 days at 37 °C until hematopoietic colonies develop. Since neutropenia is the dose-limiting effect of most cytostatic agents, we analyzed *MDR1* gene transfer into precursors of the white cell lineage, colony-forming units – granulocyte-macrophage (CFU/GM). Individual colonies were picked from methylcellulose plates, lysed, and analyzed by a provirus-specific polymerase chain reaction. Twenty to sixty percent of colonies were found to contain the proviral *MDR1* gene. P-glycoprotein function was investigated in lineage-committed progenitors following semisolid and liquid culture. Colony-forming cells were incubated with increasing concentrations of vincristine, an *MDR1*-related cytostatic agent. Following cocultivation of CD34+-selected mobilized peripheral blood progenitor cells on *MDR1* retroviral producer cells, up to 20% of CFU-GM colonies were resistant to the drug while only 1% of the mock-transduced control colonies survived, which is comparable to *MDR1* transduction data reported by others

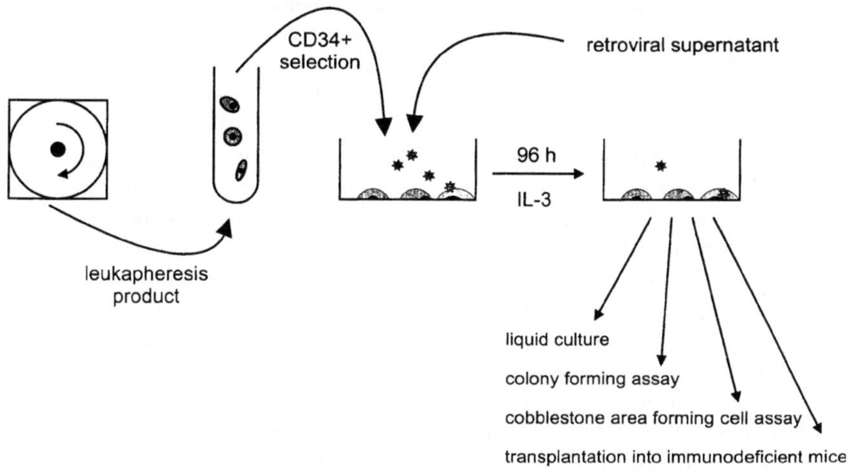

Fig. 6. The expression of the transferred *MDR*1 gene can be studied with in vitro assays for human hematopoietic stem cells or with human-mouse transplantation chimaerae

with cord blood or bone marrow as stem cell source (Bertolini et al. 1994; Boesen et al. 1995). When cell-free retroviral supernatant was used, up to 11% of CFU-GM colonies were vincristine-resistant. Interestingly, there was no difference between either IL-3 or combinations of IL-3 and SCF or IL-3/SCF and IL-6 added during *MDR*1 retroviral gene transfer with regard to the induction of cytostatic drug resistance.

Fluorescence-activated cell sorting (FACS) analysis allowed comparison of the P-glycoprotein expression on a semiquantitative scale between *MDR*1 and mock-transduced samples. CD34+ cells express low levels of P-glycoprotein while mature granulocytes and monocytes are essentially devoid of it. Therefore, we incubated the transduced CD34+ blood cells in a cytokine cocktail that leads to terminal maturation in the myelomonocytic lineage, i.e., the generation of CD15+/CD11b+ cells at the expense of the CD34+ compartment. Rhodamine-123 is a fluorescent dye and an efficient substrate of the *MDR*1 pump. Following retroviral gene transfer, 1%–5% of the cultured cells were rhodamine-123^{dull} with a median 2 log reduction in rhodamine-123 retention compared to controls, suggesting high-level *MDR*1 expression in the progeny of the transduced blood cells.

Long-term culture-initiating cells (LTCIC) are considered to be a measure of the long-term reconstitution potential of a hematopoietic graft, and expression of a gene in these cells is thought to represent long-term expression in vivo. Transfer of the *MDR*1 gene into human LTCIC from bone marrow has been demonstrated. However, for a frequency analysis, a limiting-dilution set-up is required so that Poisson can be applied. In the LTCIC assay developed by the group of Eaves in Vancouver (Sutherland et al. 1990), after 5–8 weeks culture at 33 °C, individual wells are plated in semisolid cultures and grown for another 14 days before evaluation. The recently described human cobblestone area forming cell (CAFC) assay (Breems et al. 1994) allows, in a single culture, direct enumeration of phase-contrast dark hematopoietic clones (cobblestone area) growing below the stromal layer that can be successively scored and that represent progeny of both mature and primitive precursor cells. In the mouse, the CAFC day-10 frequency is indicative of transient repopulating ability, while CAFC day 28 or later represent stem cells with long-term repopulation potential (Ploemacher 1994). In Fig. 7 a representative CAFC assay of CD34+ selected and transduced blood cells is depicted. Following *MDR*1 supernatant transduction of peripheral blood progenitor cells and culturing in the CAFC assay for 6 weeks, a large fraction of 22% of primitive week-6 cells had integrated the transduced gene in their DNA (Fruehauf et al. 1996). To screen for P-glycoprotein overexpression in *MDR*1-transduced peripheral blood progenitor cells, vincristine was added to the CAFC cultures. The mean proportion of 1% vincristine-resistant CAFC week-6 cells was comparatively low, suggesting inefficient transcriptional activation or repression of MoMLV LTRs (Challita et al. 1995; Valerio 1992). Recent results pointed to an expression-limiting viral enhancer region in the U3 region of the MoMLV LTR, which led to the construction of modified retroviral vectors that are currently being tested (Baum et al. 1995).

Transplantation of human peripheral blood progenitor cells in immune-deficient mice allows study of the repopulation potential of transduced cells as well as gene integration and expression in the various blood cell lineages (Nol-

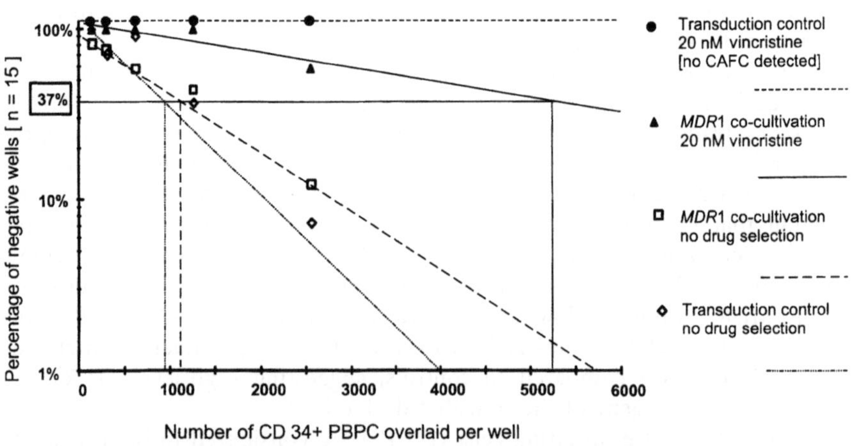

Fig. 7. Limiting-dilution analysis of CD34+ selected hematopoietic progenitor cells cocultivated on *MDR*1 vector producing irradiated packaging cells in the presence of IL-3 for 96 h. Stroma-dependent cultures were maintained for 6 weeks and cobblestone areas were counted. Percentages of negative wells at a series of input cells per well are given. The single-hit kinetics that is the basis of Poisson statistics is illustrated by the observation that linearly fitted lines extrapolate to the origin of the coordinate system. According to Poisson statistics, when 37% of wells are negative, one cobblestone area-forming cell (CAFC) is contained in a given number of cells as depicted. While the growth of *MDR*1-transduced and control cells was comparable without drug selection, in 20 n*M* vincristine only *MDR*1-transduced cells survived (controls 100% negative wells at all dilutions)

ta et al. 1995; Wermann et al. 1996; Fig. 8), which provides further valuable information before clinical application can be considered. After pretesting of several immune-deficient strains, *nonobese diabetic / severe combined immune deficiency (NOD/SCID)* mice were chosen for retroviral transduction studies as they showed reproducible multilineage engraftment following transplantation of 5×10^5 human CD 34+ cells (Wermann et al. 1996). In a manner comparable to the clinical situation, mice received radiation conditioning 24 h prior to transplantation of CD 34+-selected peripheral blood progenitor cells. The cell viability and the percentage of CD 34+ cells ranged above 90% in each sample. After grafting the human cytokines IL-3 and G-CSF were administered subcutaneously to enhance human cell engraftment. At 2 and 4 weeks after transplantation mouse peripheral blood was analyzed for the presence of mouse CD 45– and human CD 45+ leukocytes. At week 5–6 mouse bone marrow, spleen, and peripheral blood were obtained and used for the rhodamine efflux assay. Surprisingly, the threshold dose of 5×10^5 CD 34+ cells did not produce engraftment with human cells in any of the recipients when CD 34+ cells were cultured in IL-3 for 96 h, either in the transduction controls or in the *MDR* 1-supernatant or *MDR* 1-cocultivated group. Only when four times as many stem cells were transplanted did we find engraftment with up to 22% human cells following *MDR* 1-transduction (Table 1). A three-color FACS analysis for the human pan-leukocyte antigen CD 45, for mouse CD 45, and for rhodamine-123 revealed long-term reconstitution with a population of human P-gly-

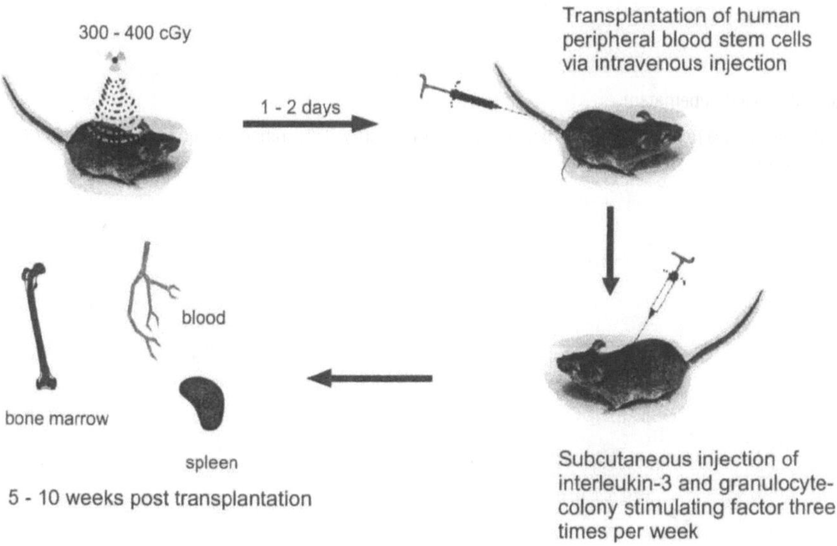

Fig. 8. In a human-mouse hematopoietic stem cell chimaera the engraftment potential of cytokine-expanded or retrovirus-transduced human stem cells can be tested in a preclinical model. In a similar way to patients, mice receive radiation conditioning therapy following intravenous transplantation. After grafting mice receive human growth factors to enhance engraftment. Eventually hematopoietic organs are analyzed for the presence of human cells

coprotein-expressing rhodamine-123^{dull} cells in the bone marrow, suggesting *MDR*1 gene transfer into repopulating stem cells (Fig. 9). Further experiments will be directed to improve the reconstitution capacity of retrovirally transduced cells, e.g., by stroma-derived factors (Conneally et al. 1996; Nolta et al. 1995), and to increase the transduction efficiency by optimization of virus harvesting and transduction protocols as described.

Alternatives to Retroviral Vectors

In contrast to retroviral vectors, adenoviruses and adeno-associated viruses (AAV) (see Ogniben and Haas, this volume) are able to infect growth-arrested

Table 1. Transplantation of human CD34+ selected peripheral blood progenitor cells (PBPC) transduced with *MDR*1 for 96 h in the presence of IL-3 into NOD/SCID mice

Compartment	Engraftment period	Number of mice repopulating with human CD45+ leukocytes			
		Control	*MDR*1-SNT	*MDR*1 cocultivated	
		5×10^5/graft[a]	5×10^5/graft[a]	5×10^5/graft[a]	2×10^6/graft[a]
	Week 2	0/2	2/4	2/3	3/3
Peripheral blood	Week 4	2/2	1/4	0/2	3/3
	Week 5	0/1	0/4	0/2	3/3
Bone marrow	Week 5	0/1	0/4	0/2	3/3
Spleen	Week 5	0/1	0/4	0/2	2/3

SNT, Retroviral supernatant.

[a] Number of CD34+ PBPC grafted per mouse; CD34+ purity 91%; range of human CD45+ leukocytes >0.1%–21.9%.

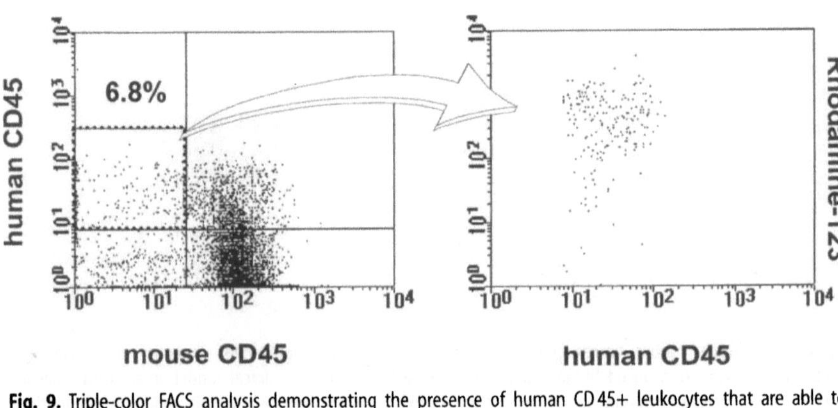

Fig. 9. Triple-color FACS analysis demonstrating the presence of human CD45+ leukocytes that are able to exclude the fluorescent dye rhodamine-123 following retroviral *MDR*1 transduction of human CD34+ peripheral blood progenitor cells and transplantation in immune-deficient mice

cells (Alexander et al. 1994). Adenovirus remains episomal, with occasional integration, while AAV is able to integrate stably into the genome (Fisher-Adams et al. 1996). The genes transferred with the AAV system so far include the Fanconi anemia complementation group C gene, the γ-globin gene into human erythroid colony-forming cells and the human *MDR*1 gene. Since the complete *MDR*1 gene is too large for use in AAV vectors, the minimal open reading frame (ORF) of the gene driven by the Rous sarcoma virus LTR was used, which is altogether about 200 bp larger than the wild-type AAV genome but could still be packaged efficiently (Fisher-Adams et al. 1996). The gene transfer frequency ranged from 20% to 80% in various studies (Miller et al. 1994; Shaughnessy et al. 1996; Walsh et al. 1994; Zhou et al. 1993) which would be comparable to retrovirus vectors. However, it should be borne in mind that AAV is a stable DNA particle which may have entered a progenitor cell without integratintg into its genome, so positive PCR results may overestimate the true efficiency of transduction. Functional studies are required for comparison.

Future Perspectives

Somatic gene transfer in conjunction with hematopoietic stem cell transplantation will gain clinical relevance in the forthcoming years. Current gene-marking protocols will allow conclusions to be drawn about the relevance of purging methods and the conditions for efficient gene transfer to hematopoietic cells. The transfer of drug resistance genes will gain importance if it becomes possible to achieve meaningful myeloprotection during chemotherapy. Furthermore, insights into the selection possibilities of transduced cells in vivo and the level and duration of expression will allow the drawing of conclusions which also bear on nononcological gene therapy applications. The careful selection of suitable genes of interest, vectors, and transduction protocols are decisive parameters for the efficacy and biological safety of gene therapeutic strategies. Only systematic analysis and further development in all fields of gene transfer will ultimately lead to a successful application in oncology.

Acknowledgments. This work was supported by a grant of the Deutsche Krebshilfe/Mildred-Scheel Stiftung. The authors are grateful to helpful suggestions made by Dr. B. Schiedlmeier.

References

Alexander IE, Russel DW, Miller AD (1994) DNA-damaging agents greatly increase the transduction of non-dividing cells by adeno-associated virus vectors. J Virol 68:8282–8287

Allay JA, Dumenco LL, Koc ON, Liu L, Gerson SL (1995) Retroviral transduction and expression of the human alkyltransferase cDNA provides nitrosourea resistance to hematopoietic cells. Blood 85:3342–3351

Anderson WF, McGarrity GJ, Moen RC (1993) Report to the NIH recombinant DNA advisory committee on murine replication-competent retrovirus (RCR) assay. Hum Gene Ther 4:311–321

Baum C, Ostertag W (1996) Somatischer Gentransfer in der Onkologie. In: Zeller WJ, zur Hausen H (eds) Onkologie. Grundlagen, Diagnostik, Therapie, Entwicklungen. Ecomed, Landsberg, pp 1–23

Baum C, Hegewisch-Becker S, Eckert HG, Stocking C, Ostertag W (1995) Novel retroviral vectors for efficient expression of the multidrug resistance (*mdr*-1) gene in early hematopoietic cells. J Virol 69:7541–7547

Berenson RJ, Andrews RG, Bensinger WI, Kalamasz D, Knitter G, Buckner CD, Bernstein ID (1988) Antigen CD34+ marrow cells engraft lethally irradiated baboons. J Clin Invest 81:951–955

Berenson RJ, Bensinger WI, Hill RS, Andrews RG, Garcia-Lopez J, Kalamasz DF, Still BJ, Spitzer G, Buckner CD, Bernstein ID, Thomas ED (1991) Engraftment after infusion of CD34+ marrow cells in patients with breast cancer or neuroblastoma. Blood 77:1717–1722

Bertolini F, de Monte L, Corsini C, Lazzari L, Lauri E, Soligo D, Ward M, Bank A, Malavasi F (1994) Retrovirus-mediated transfer of the multidrug resistance gene into human haemopoietic progenitor cells. Br J Haematol 88:318–324

Bertolini F, Battaglia M, Corsini C, Lazzari L, Soligo D, Zibero C, Thalmeier K (1996) Engineered stromal layers and continuous flow culture enhance multidrug resistance gene transfer in hematopoietic progenitors. Cancer Res 56:2566–2572

Boesen J, Brouwer K, Hospers G, Nooter K, Valerio D (1995) Introduction of the *MDR* 1 gene into hematopoietic stem cells to improve cancer chemotherapy. In: Zeller WJ, Eisenbrand G, Hellman K (eds) Reduction of anticancer drug toxicity. Pharmacologic, biologic, immunologic and gene therapeutic approaches. Karger, Basel, pp 118–124 (contributions to oncology, vol 48)

Breems DA, Blokland EAW, Neben S, Ploemacher RE (1995) Frequency analysis of human primitive haematopoietic cell assay. Leukemia 8:1095–1104

Brenner MK, Rill DR, Moen RC, Krance RA, Mirro J Jr, Anderson WF, Ihle JN (1993) Gene marking to trace origin of relapse after autologous bone marrow transplantation. Lancet 341:85–86

Bunnell BA, Muul LM, Donahue RE, Blaese RM, Morgan RA (1995) High-efficiency retroviral-mediated gene transfer into human and non-human primate peripheral blood lymphocytes. Proc Natl Acad Sci USA 92:7739–7743

Challita PM, Skelton D, El Khouery A, Yu XJ, Weinberg K, Kohn DB (1995) Multiple modifications in cis elements of the long terminal repeat of retroviral vectors lead to increased expression and decreased DNA methylation in embryonic carcinoma cells. J Virol 69:748–755

Chuck AS, Palsson BO (1996) Consistent and high rates of gene transfer can be obtained using flow-through transduction over a wide range of retroviral titers. Hum Gene Ther 7:743–750

Civin CI, Strauss LC, Brovall C, Fackler MJ, Schwartz JF, Shaper JH (1984) Antigenic analysis of hematopoiesis. A hematopoietic progenitor cell surface antigen defined by a monoclonal antibody raised against KG-1a cells. J Immunol 133:157–165

Civin CI, Strauss LC, Fackler MJ, Trischmann TM, Wiley JM, Loken MR (1990) Positive stem cell selection – basic science. Prog Clin Biol Res 333:387–401

Conneally E, Eaves CJ, Humphries RK (1996) High efficiency gene transfer to primitive human hematopoietic cells capable of multilineage repopulation of immunodeficient *NOD/SCID* mice. Blood 88 Suppl 1:646a

Cornetta K, Nguyen N, Morgan RA, Muenchau DD, Hartley JW, Blaese RM, Anderson WF (1993) Infection of human cells with murine amphotropic replication-competent retroviruses. Hum Gene Ther 4:579–588

Cosset FL, Morling FJ, Takeuchi Y, Weiss RA, Collins MK, Russell SJ (1995) Retroviral retargeting by envelopes expressing a N-terminal binding domain. J Virol 69:6314–6322

Crooks GM, Kohn DB (1993) Growth factors increase amphotropic retrovirus binding to human CD34+ bone marrow progenitor cells. Blood 82:3290–3297

Danos O, Mulligan RC (1988) Safe and efficient generation of recombinant retroviruses with amphotropic and ecotropic host ranges. Proc Natl Acad Sci USA 85:6460–6464

Deisseroth AB, Zu Z, Claxton D, Hanania EG, Fu S, Ellerson D, Goldberg L, Thomas M, Janicek K, Anderson WJ, Hester J, Korbling M, Durett A, Moen R, Berenson R, Heimfeld S, Hamer J, Calvert L, Tibbits P, Talpaz M, Kantarjian H, Champlin R, Reading C (1994) Genetic marking shows that Ph+ cells present in autologous transplants of chronic myelogenous leukemia (CML) contribute to relapse after autologous bone marrow transplantation in CML. Blood 83:3068–3076

Dirks W, Wirth M, Hauser H (1993) Dicistronic transcription units for gene expression in mammalian cells. Gene 128:247–249

Donahue RE, Kessler SW, Bodine D, McDonagh K, Dunbar C, Goodman S, Agricola B, Byrne E, Raffeld M, Moen R, Bacher J, Zsebo KM, Nienhuis AW (1992) Helper virus induced T cell lymphoma in non-human primates after retroviral mediated gene transfer. J Exp Med 176:1125–1135

Dunbar CE, Dottler-Fox M, O'Shaughnessy JA, Doren S, Carter C, Berenson R, Brown S, Moen RC, Greenblatt J, Stewart FM, Leitman SF, Wyndham JW, Cowan K, Young NS, Nienhuis AW (1995) Retrovirally marked CD34-enriched peripheral blood and bone marrow cells contribute to long-term engraftment after autologous transplantation. Blood 85:3048–3057

Dunbar CE, Seidel NE, Doren S, Sellers S, Cline AP, Metzger ME, Agricola BA, Donahue RE, Bodine DM (1996) Improved retroviral gene transfer into murine and rhesus peripheral blood or bone marrow repopulating cells primed in vivo with stem cell factor and granulocyte colony stimulating factor. Proc Natl Acad Sci USA 93:11871–11876

Dybing J, Lynch C, Hara P, Leonard J, Anklesaria P (1995) GALV pseudotyped vectors transduce human bone marrow CD34+ $CD38^{lo}$ cells with high efficiency. Blood 86 Suppl 1:3975

Eckert HG, Stockschläder M, Just U, Hegewisch-Becker S, Grez M, Uhde A, Zander A, Ostertag W, Baum C (1996) High-dose multidrug resistance in primary human hematopoietic progenitor cells transduced with optimizing retroviral vectors. Blood 88:3407–3415

Emerman M, Temin HM (1986) Comparison of promoter suppression in avian and murine retrovirus vectors. Nucleic Acids Res 14:9381–9386

Faustinella F, Kwon H, Serrano F, Belmont JW, Caskey CT, Aguilar-Cordova E (1994) A new family of retroviral fectors with extended multiple cloning sites for gene insertion. Hum Gene Ther 5:307–312

Fisher-Adams G, Wong KK, Podsakoff G, Forman SJ, Chatterjee S (1996) Integration of adeno-associated virus vectors in CD34+ human hematopoietic progenitor cells after transduction. Blood 88:492–504

Flasshove M, Banerjee D, Minesishi S, Li MX, Bertino JR, Moore MAS (1995) Ex vivo expansion and selection of human CD34+ peripheral blood progenitor cells after introduction of a mutated dihydrofolate reductase cDNA via retroviral gene transfer. Blood 85:566–574

Fruehauf S, Haas R, Zeller WJ, Hunstein W (1994) CD34 selection for purging in multiple myeloma and analysis of CD34+ B cell precursors. Stem Cells 12:95–102

Fruehauf S, Breems DA, Knaän-Shanzer S, Brouwer KB, Haas R, Löwenberg B, Nooter K, Ploemacher RE, Valerio D, Boesen JB (1996) Frequency analysis of multidrug resistance-1 gene transfer into human primitive hematopoietic progenitor cells using the cobblestone area forming cell assay and detection of fector-mediated P-glycoprotein expression by rhodamine-123. Hum Gene Ther 7:1219–1231

Galski H, Sullivan M, Willingham MC, Chin KV, Gottesman MM, Pastan I, Merlino GT (1989) Expression of a human multidrug resistance cDNA (*MDR*1) in the bone marrow of transgenic mice: resistance to daunomycin-induced leukopenia. Mol Cell Biol 9:4357–4363

Greenbaum M, Letourneau S, Assar H, Schecter RL, Batist G, Cournoyer D (1994) Retrovirus-mediated gene transfer of rat glutathione S-transferase Yc confers alkylating drug resistance in NIH 3T3 mouse fibroblasts. Cancer Res 54:4442–4447

Haas R, Mohle R, Fruehauf S, Goldschmidt H, Witt B, Flentje M, Wannenmacher M, Hunstein W (1994) Patient characteristics associated with successful mobilizing and autografting of peripheral blood progenitor cells in malignant lymphoma. Blood 83:3787–3794

Hanania EG, Fu S, Hegewisch-Becker S, Korbling M, Hester J, Durett A, Andreeff M, Mechtner E, Holzmeyer T, Roninson IB, Giles RE, Berenson R, Heimfeld S, Deisseroth AB (1995) Chemotherapy resistance to taxol in clonogenic progenitor cells following transduction of CD34 selected marrows and peripheral blood cells with a retrovirus that contains the *MDR*1 chemotherapy resistance gene. Gene Ther 2:285–294

Hanenberg H, Yiao XL, Dilloo D, Hashino K, Kato I, Williams DA (1996) Colocalization of retrovirus and target cells on specific fibronectin fragments increases genetic transduction of mammalian cells. Nature Med 2:876–882

Hanley ME, Nolta JA, Parkman R, Kohn DB (1994) Umbilical cord blood cell transduction by retroviral vectors: preclinical studies to optimize gene transfer. Blood Cells 20:539–546

Hoogerbrugge PM, Vossen JM, van Beusechem VW, Valerio D (1992) Treatment of patients with severe combined immunodeficiency due to adenosine deaminase (ADA) by autologous transplantation of genetically modified bone marrow cells. Hum Gene Ther 3:553–558

Hughes PF, Thacker JD, Hogge D, Sutherland HJ, Thomas TE, Lansdorp PM, Eaves CJ, Humphries RK (1992) Retroviral gene transfer to primitive normal and leukemic hematopoietic cells using clinically applicable procedures. J Clin Invest 89:1817–1824

Jolly D (1994) Viral vector systems for gene therapy. Cancer Gene Ther 1:51–64

Kiem HP, Darovsky B, von Kalle C, Goehle S, Steward D, Graham T, Hackman R, Appelbaum FR, Deeg J, Miller AD, Storb R, Schuening FG (1994) Retrovirus-mediated gene transduction into canine peripheral blood repopulating cells. Blood 83:1467–1473

Kodama H, Sudo H, Koyama H, Kasai S, Yamamoto S (1984) In vitro hemopoiesis within a microenvironment created by MC3T3-G2/PA6 preadipocytes. J Cell Physiol 118:233–240

Koo HM, Brown AMC, Kaufman RJ, Prorock CM, Ron Y, Dougherty JP (1992) A spleen necrosis virus-based retroviral vector which expresses two genes from a dicistronic mRNA. Virology 186:669–675

Kotani H, Newton PB, Zhang S, Chiang YL, Otto E, Weaver L, Blaese M, Anderson F, McGarrity GJ (1994) Improved methods of retroviral vector transduction and production for gene therapy. Hum Gene Ther 5:19–28

Kozak SL, Siess DC, Kavanaugh MP, Miller AD, Kabat D (1995) The envelope glycoprotein of an amphotropic murine retrovirus binds specifically to the cellular receptor/phosphate transporter of susceptible species. J Virol 69:3433–3440

Levine F, Yee JK, Friedmann T (1991) Efficient gene expression in mammalian cells from a dicistronic transcriptional unit in an improved retroviral vector. Gene 108:167–174

Lewis P, Hensel M, Emerman M (1992) Human immunodeficiency virus infection of cells arrested in the cell cycle. EMBO J 11:3053–3058

Li MX, Banerjee D, Zhao SC, Schweitzer BI, Mineishi S, Gilboa E, Bertino JR (1994) Development of a retroviral construct containing a human mutated dihydrofolate reductase cDNA for hematopoietic stem cell transduction. Blood 83:3403–3408

Lieber A, Vrancken Peeters MJTFD, Kay M (1995) Adenovirus-mediated transfer of the amphotropic retrovirus receptor cDNA increases retroviral transduction in cultured cells. Hum Gene Ther 6:5–11

Lu M, Maruyama M, Zhang N, Levine F, Friedman T, Ho AD (1994) High efficiency retroviral-mediated gene transduction into CD34+ cells purified from peripheral blood of breast cancer patients primed with chemotherapy and granulocyte-macrophage colony-stimulating factor. Hum Gene Ther 5:203–208

Magni M, Shammah S, Schiro R, Mellado W, Dalla-Favera R, Gianni AM (1996) Introduction of cyclophosphamide resistance by aldehyde dehydrogenase-1 gene transfer. Blood 87:1097–1103

Markowitz D, Goff S, Bank A (1988a) A safe packaging line for gene transfer: separating viral genes on two different plasmids. J Virol 62:1120–1124

Markowitz D, Goff S, Bank A (1988b) Construction and use of a safe and efficient amphotropic packaging cell line. Virology 167:400–406

Metz MZ, Matsumoto L, Winters KA, Doroshow JH, Kane SE (1996) Bicistronic and two-gene retroviral vectors for using mdr1 as a selectable marker and a therapeutic gene. Virology 217:230–241

Miller AD, Buttimore C (1986) Redesign of retrovirus packaging cell lines to avoid recombination leading to helper virus production. Mol Cell Biol 6:2895–2902

Miller AD, Chen F (1996) Retrovirus packaging cells based on 10A1 murine leukemia virus for production of vectors that use multiple receptors for cell entry. J Virol 70:5564–5571

Miller AD, Garcia JV, von Suhr N, Lynch CM, Wilson C, von Eiden M (1991) Construction and properties of packaging cells based on gibbon ape leukemia virus. J Virol 65:2220–2224

Miller DG, Miller AD (1994) A family of retroviruses that utilize related phosphate transporters for cell entry. J Virol 68:8270–8276

Miller JL, Donahue RE, Sellers SE, Samulski RJ, Young NS, Nienhuis AW (1994) Recombinant adeno-associated virus (rAAV)-mediated expression of a human gamma-globin gene in human progenitor-derived erythroid cells. Proc Natl Acad Sci USA 91:10183–10187. [Erratum in Proc Natl Acad Sci USA (1995) 92:646]

Miller N, Vile R (1995) Targeted vectors for gene therapy. FASEB J 9:190–199

Mitani K, Graham FL, Caskey CT (1994) Transduction of human bone marrow by adenoviral vector. Hum Gene Ther 5:941–948

Moore KA, Deisseroth AB, Reading CL, Williams DE, Belmont JW (1992) Stromal support enhances cell-free retroviral vector transduction of human bone marrow long-term culture-initiating cells. Blood 79:1393–1399

Morgan RA, Couture L, Elroy-Stein O, Ragheb J, Moss B, Anderson WF (1992) Retroviral vectors containing putative internal ribosome entry sites: development of a polycistronic gene transfer system and applications to human gene therapy. Nucleic Acids Res 20:1293–1299

Moritz T, Patel VP, Williams DA (1994) Bone marrow extracellular matrix molecules improve gene transfer into human hematopoietic cells via retroviral vectors. J Clin Invest 93:1451–1457

Moritz T, Dutt P, Xiao X, Carstanjen D, Vik T, Hanenberg H, Williams DA (1996) Fibronectin improves transduction of reconstituting hematopoietic stem cells by retroviral vectors: evidence of direct viral binding to chymotryptic carboxy-terminal fragments. Blood 88:855–862

Naldini L, Blömer U, Gallay P, Ory D, Mulligan R, Gage FH, Verma IM, Trono D (1996) In vivo gene delivery and stable transduction of nondividing cells by a lentiviral vector. Science 272:263–267

Nolta JA, Smorgorzewska EM, Kohn DB (1995) Analysis of optimal conditions of retrovira-mediated transduction of primitive human hematopoietic cells. Blood 86:101–110

Orlic D, Girard LJ, Craig TJ, Anderson SM, Cline AP, Bodine DM (1996) The level of mRNA encoding the amphotropic retrovirus receptor in mouse and human hematopoietic stem cells is low and correlates with the efficiency to retrovirus transduction. Proc Natl Acad Sci USA 93:11097–11102

Palsson BO, Chuck AS, Huang G (1995) Retroviral infection is limited by random brownian motion. Blood 86 Suppl 1:933

Paul RW, Morris D, Hess BW, Dunn J, Overell RW (1993) Increased viral titer through concentration of viral harvests from retroviral packaging lines. Hum Gene Ther 4:609–615

Ploemacher RE (1994) Cobblestone area forming cell (CAFC) assay. In: Freshney RI, Pragnell IB, Freshney MG (eds) Culture of hematopoietic cells. Wiley-Liss, New York, pp 1–21

Pulsipher M, Guitierrez-Ramos JC, Friedrich C, Mulligan RC, Nathan DG, Sieff CA (1995) A murine stromal cell line engineered to express human IL-3 enhances retroviral-mediated gene transfer. Blood 86 Suppl 1:1626

Russ AP, Friedel C, Grez M, Melchner HV (1996) Self-deleting retrovirus vectors for gene therapy. J Virol 70:4927–4932

Russell SJ (1996) Peptide-displaying phages for targeted gene delivery. Nat Med 2:276–277

Salmons B, Günzburg WH (1993) Targeting of retroviral vectors for gene therapy. Hum Gene Ther 4:129–141

Salmons B, Saller RM, Baumann JG, Günzburg W (1995) Construction of retroviral vectors for targeted delivery and expression of therapeutic genes. Leukemia 9:53–60

Samson LD (1992) The repair of DNA alkylation damage by methyltransferases and glycosylases. Essays Biochem 27:69–78

Schuening FG, Storb R, Meyer J, Jaehle S (1989) Long term culture of canine bone marrow cells. Exp Haematol 17:411–417

Sekhar M, Prentice HG, MacDonald I, McGarrity G, Foroni L, Yong K (1995) Retroviral transduction of CD34-enriched haematopoietic progenitor cells in the presence of an endothelial monolayer. Blood 86 Suppl 1:1008

Shaughnessy E, Lu D, Chatterjee S, Wong KK (1996) Parvoviral vectors for gene therapy of cancer. Semin Oncol 23:159–171

Shi YJ, Shen RN, Lu L, Broxmeyer HE (1994) Comparative analysis of retroviral-mediated gene transduction into CD34+ cord blood hematopoietic progenitors in the presence and absence of growth factors. Blood Cells 20:517–524

Sorrentino BP, Brand SJ, Bodine D, Gottesman MM, Pastan I, Cline A, Nienhuis AW (1992) Selection of drug-resistant bone marrow cells in vivo after retroviral transfer of human. *MDR* 1. Science 257:99–103

Sorrentino BP, McDonagh KT, Woods D, Orlic D (1995) Expression of retroviral vectors containing the human multidrug-resistance 1 cDNA in hematopoietic cells of transplanted mice. Blood 86:491–501

Sugimoto Y, Aksentijevich I, Gottesman MM, Pastan I (1994) Efficient expression of drug-selectable genes in retroviral vectors under control of an internal ribosomal entry site. Biotechnology 12:694–698

Sutherland HJ, Lansdorp PM, Henkelman DH, Eaves AC, Eaves CJ (1990) Functional characterization of individual human hematopoietic stem cells cultured at limiting dilution on supportive marrow stromal layers. Proc Natl Acad Sci USA 87:3584–3588

Torrent C, Berlioz C, Darlix JL (1996) Stable MLV-VL30 dicistronic retroviral vectors with a VL30 or MoMLV sequence promoting both packaging of genomid RNA and expression of the 3' cistron. Hum Gene Ther 7:603–612

Uckert W, Walther W (1994) Retrovirus-mediated gene transfer in cancer therapy. Pharmacol Ther 63:323–347

Valerio D (1992) Retrovirus vectors for gene therapy procedures. In: Grosveld F, Kollias G (eds) Transgenic mice in biology and medicine. Academic, London, pp 211–246

Van Beusechem VW, Kuhler A, Heidt PJ, Valerio D (1992) Long-term expression of human adenosine deaminase in rhesus monkeys transplanted with retrovirus infected bone marrow cells. Proc Natl Acad Sci USA 89:7640–7644

Van Beusechem VW, Bakx TA, Kaptein LCM, Bart-Baumeister JAK, Kukler A, Braakman E, Valerio D (1993) Retrovirus-mediated gene transfer into rhesus monkey hematopoietic stem cells: the effect of viral titers on transduction efficiency. Hum Gene Ther 4:239–247

Van Germeraad WTV, Asami N, Fujimoto S, Mazda O, Katsura Y (1994) Efficient retrovirus gene transduction into murine hematopoietic stem cells and long-lasting expression using a transwell coculture system. Blood 84:780–788

Von Kalle C, Kiem HP, Goehle S, Darovsky B, Heimfield S, Torok-Storb B, Storb R, Schuening FG (1994) Increased gene transfer into human hematopoietic progenitor cells by extended in vitro exposure to a pseudotyped retroviral vector. Blood 84:2890–2897

Walsh CE, Nienhuis AW, Samulski RJ, Brown MG, Miller JL, Young NS, Liu JM (1994) Phenotypic correction of Fanconi anemia in human hematopoietic cells with a recombinant adeno-associated virus vector. J Clin Invest 94:1440–1448

Ward M, Richarson C, Pioli P, Smith L, Podda S, Goff S, Hesdorffer C, Bank A (1994) Transfer and expression of the human multiple drug resistance gene in human CD34+ cells. Blood 84:1408–1414

Webb M, Sorrentino BP (1994) Retroviral transfer of the human cytosolic aldehyde dehydrogenase gene as a means to generate cellular cyclophosphamide resistance. Blood 84 Suppl 1:357a

Weiss RA, Tailor CS (1995) Retrovirus receptors. Cell 82:531–533

Wermann K, Fruehauf S, Haas R, Zeller WJ (1996) Human-mouse xenografts in stem cell research. Hematother 5:379–390

Xu LC, Young HA, Blanco M, Kessler S, Roberts AB, Karlsson S (1994) Poor transduction efficiency of human hematopoietic progenitor cells by a high-titer amphotropic retrovirus producer cell clone. J Virol 68:7634–7636

Xu LC, Kluepfel-Stahl S, Blanco M, Schiffman R, Dunbar C, Karlsson S (1995) Growth factors and stromal support generate very efficient retroviral transduction of peripheral blood CD34+ cells from Gaucher patients. Blood 86:141–146

Zhou SZ, Broxmeyer HE, Cooper S, Harrington MA, Srivastava A (1993) Adeno-associated virus 2-mediated gene transfer in murine hematopoietic progenitor cells. Exp Hematol 21:928–993

Regulated Gene Expression After Retroviral Vector-Mediated Delivery of Cancer-Relevant Therapeutic Genes

W. H. Günzburg[1,2], P. Karle[1,2], S. Mrochen[1], G. Sparmann[3], R. Saller[1,5], D. Klein[2,5], W. Uckert[4], and B. Salmons[5]

[1] Institute for Molecular Virology, GSF Centre for Environmental and Health Research, 85764 Oberschleissheim, Germany
[2] Institute of Virology, University of Veterinary Medicine, Josef-Baumann-Gasse 1, 1210 Vienna, Austria
[3] Department of Gastroenterology, Rostock University, 18057 Rostock, Germany
[4] Max Delbruck Centre, 13125 Berlin-Buck, Germany
[5] Bavarian Nordic Research Institute, 85764 Oberschleissheim, Germany

Introduction

The transfer of therapeutic genes to cells, a concept known as gene therapy, promises to provide a new, more focussed assault on a wide range of diseases, including solid tumours and leukaemias. Cancer is thought to arise as a consequence of the accumulation of multiple genetic lesions and at some stage the process becomes irreversible (Ewald et al. 1996). This suggests that this group of diseases cannot be treated by classical gene augmentation therapy as has been used for monogenetic disorders. A number of approaches have been taken towards the elimination of tumour cells using gene therapy. Here the potential application of some of these tumour therapy relevant genes are discussed with the aim of using retrovirus vectors as the gene transfer system to deliver these therapeutic genes.

Retroviral Vectors as Gene Delivery Systems

A number of methods have been developed for gene transfer purposes, including physical methods such as transfection, lipofection, electroporation and even biolistics, in which DNA-coated particles are shot into cells using a "gene gun" (reviewed in Günzburg and Salmons 1996). However, more efficient delivery systems have been derived from naturally occurring gene transfer agents, the viruses. Retroviruses, adenoviruses, adeno-associated viruses and herpes viruses have all been genetically manipulated to create gene transfer or vector systems, with more systems derived from other viruses planned (Günzburg, and Salmons 1995, 1996). Retroviral vectors are by far the most commonly used of all gene transfer systems, whether physical or viral, in human gene therapy trials (Herrmann 1996). A major concern, particularly for gene therapy of cancer, is the ability to deliver genes to

Recent Results in Cancer Research, Vol. 144

and express the therapeutic gene in target (tumour) cells and not in other cells – this is especially important if the therapeutic gene encodes a product that is either toxic or confers drug-mediated cytotoxicity (suicide) on the recipient and surrounding cells. Recently we have developed a new type of retroviral vector in which expression of the therapeutic gene is driven from a heterologous promoter of choice (Salmons et al. 1995; Saller et al. 1997) (Fig. 1). Promoters of interest include those that are regulatable or active specifically in tumour cells. Since the heterologous promoter replaces that of the retrovirus, these vectors have been termed "promoter conversion" (ProCon) vectors. Replacement of the promoter prevents the phenomenon of promoter interference that may affect promoter specificity and function and may also contribure to the safety of these vectors (Saller et al. 1997).

Cancer-Relevant Therapeutic Genes

Gene therapy promises to be a powerful means to treat cancer and this is reflected by the fact that over 50% of the ongoing clinical trials are directed at cancer (Hermann 1996). These trials are all based upon encouraging results obtained in animal cancer models.

The therapeutic genes and strategies that have been used include 1) enhancement of immune responses to the tumour (see Westermann et al. and Meuer et al.; this volume), 2) inhibition of cell growth (see Kronenwett and Haas, this volume), 3) introduction and expression of tumour suppressor genes and 4) expression of genes encoding either toxic gene products or products that activate a prodrug, all of which are discussed below.

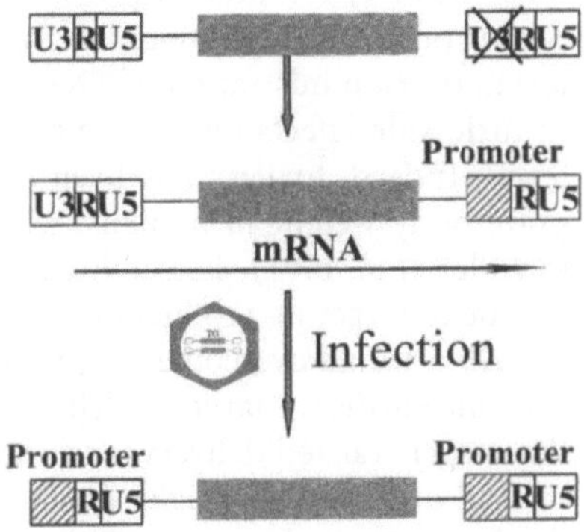

Fig. 1. The ProCon (promoter conversion) retroviral vector. The U3 region within the 3′ long terminal repeat (LTR) (U3-R-U5) of a retroviral vector carrying a therapeutic gene (*shaded box*) is deleted and replaced with a heterologous promoter (*hatched box*). In the packaging cell line, expression of the retroviral vector mRNA is driven by the normal retroviral promoter located within the U3 region of the 5′LTR. This RNA, which initiates at the junction between the U3 and R regions of the 5′LTR, and terminates between the R and U5 region of the 3′LTR, is packaged into the recombinant viral particle. After infection this RNA is reverse transcribed in the target cell, as a result of which the heterologous promoter in the 3′LTR becomes duplicated and placed at both ends of the resulting proviral structure. In the target cell, expression of the therapeutic gene is then controlled by the heterologous promoter

Other strategies include reversion of the transformed phenotype and protection of non-tumour cells from the effects of conventional cancer treatments. This latter approach is of particular relevance for the protection of normal haematopoietic cells during therapy for leukaemia, where the multidrug resistance gene has been used for this purpose (Baum et al. 1995, see also Fruehauf et al., this volume).

Cytokines as a Means to Stimulate Anti-tumour Immune Responses

Cytokines are proteins that are involved in the regulation of cell proliferation and function. Lymphokines such as interleukins (ILs) are cytokines that are required specifically for activation of cells of the immune system, and IL-2, among other ILs, has been used to enhance the host immune response against tumour cells. This has involved the genetic modification of cells in the vicinity of the tumour to overexpress the lymphokine (Colombi and Forni 1994). Although this kind of approach has met with some success, one problem is that in order to elicit good activation of the immune system it appears to require the concerted action of groups of lymphokines in a series of progressive waves. Simple overexpression of one cytokine may thus not be sufficient to elicit an appropriate immune response.

Tumour necrosis factor-α (TNF-α) was the first cytokine to be used in a gene therapy trial (Rosenberg 1991). As its name implies, it has direct cytocidal or cytostatic activity against a variety of tumour cells in culture (Israel 1993). TNF-α is also a lymphokine, is produced by macrophages and can be induced in NK, T and tumour cells. The gene encoding TNF-α is located on human chromosome 6. TNF-α protein consists of 157 amino acids, the active form being a trimer of the 17-kDa subunits. Even though TNF-α is a powerful anti-cancer agent, the administration of TNF-α to cancer patients in clinical trials resulted in toxic side effects due to the high dosages required to maintain therapeutic levels. Indeed, toxicity has been observed at concentrations of 8 μg per kilogram body weight in humans, whereas mice can tolerate much higher doses (Schiller et al. 1991). The ability to target either the delivery of the TNF-α protein or to target its production to predefined cell types to give local high levels of TNF-α would overcome the problem associated with systemic delivery of the protein. Further, a targeted delivery of TNF-α may be more clinically effective than a generalized delivery, and expression systems that allow the modulation of TNF-α expression might also be beneficial. The promoter contained within the long terminal repeat (LTR) of mouse mammary tumour virus (MMTV) shows increased activity in the presence of glucocorticoid hormones such as dexamethasone and has often been used as a conditional expression system (for a review see Günzburg and Salmons 1992). In a model system, we have inserted a cDNA encoding human TNF-α (hTNF-α) into an MMTV-based retroviral vector construct (Salmons et al. 1990) in such a way as to place it under the transcriptional control of the glucocorticoid hormone responsive promoter (Fig. 2) contained within the MMTV LTR (Sparmann et al. 1994). The vector was introduced into a human glioblastoma derived cell line, U 343 MG and stable cell clones isolated. Glioblastoma cells carrying the construct showed enhanced expression of hTNF-α when grown in the presence of dexamethasone (Sparmann et al. 1994). The level of hTNF-α expressed in the presence of dexamethasone ($\sim$1.25 ng/ml) was sufficient to inhibit cell proliferation and lead to a dramatic alteration in the morphology of these cells (Fig. 3). This study demonstrates the feasibility of such an inducible approach for gene therapy. In the future, TNF-α may be placed under the transcriptional control of conditional promoters using promoter conversion retroviral vectors which are based on murine leukaemia virus (MLV) (Saller et al. 1997) (see above). MLV based retroviral vectors can only infect actively replicating cells (Miller et al. 1990), which may also be useful for targeting rapidly proliferating tumour cells.

Cell Cycle Regulators

The cell cycle regulatory protein, p21, has been shown to be overexpressed in senescent and quiescent cells or in cultured primary cells undergoing crisis (Noda et al. 1994), suggesting a role in the maintenance of DNA synthesis inhibition (Johnson et al. 1994). The direct involvement of this protein in growth inhibition has been shown by microinjection of young, actively dividing cells with a senescent cell-derived inhibitor (SDI) expression vector (Noda et al. 1994). The $p21^{SDI}$ protein prevents DNA synthesis and inhibits cell proliferation by inhibiting cyclin dependent kinase activity (Gu et al. 1993; Harper et al. 1993; Xiong et al. 1993; Nakanishi et al. 1995). Independently it has been

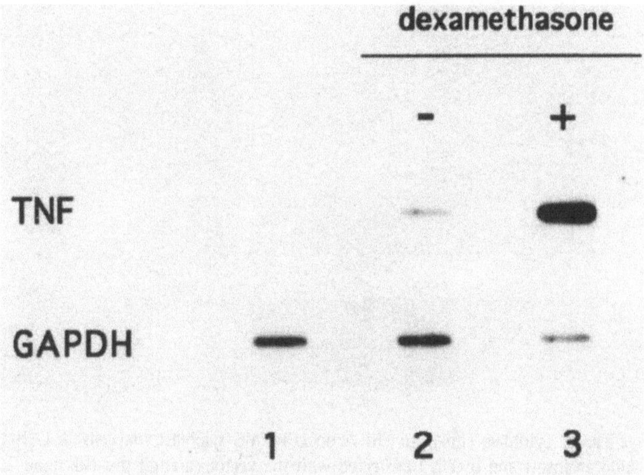

Fig. 2. Induction of TNF-α expression by dexamethasone. Shown are equivalent amounts of RNA isolated from nontransfected cells (*1*) or cells transfected with pWG29 del3-hTNF (*2, 3*) grown in the absence (*2*) or presence (*3*) of dexamethasone and hybridized to a TNF of GAPDH probe

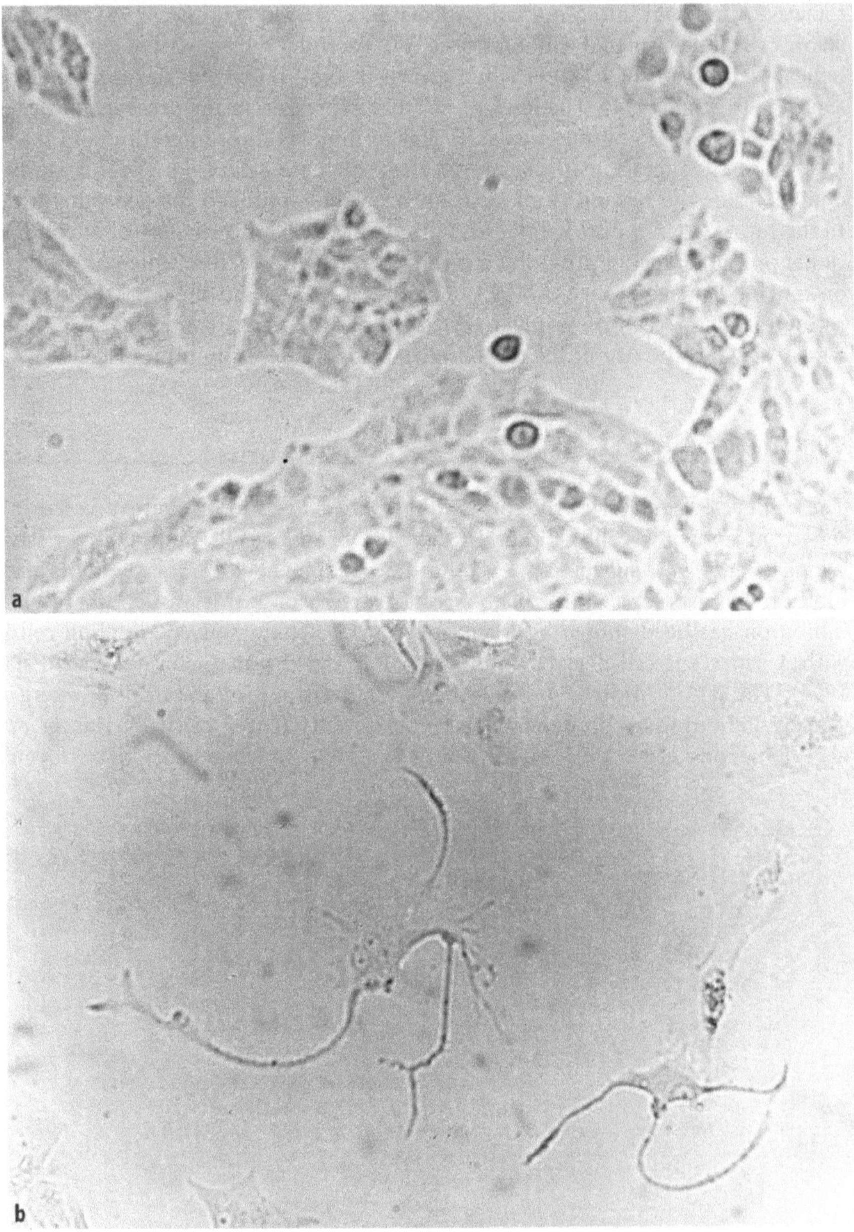

Fig. 3 a, b. Cytotoxic effects of TNF-α on U343MG glioblastoma cells. **a** Cells transfected with the vector lacking an insert and **b** cells transfected with the vector carrying the TNF gene

shown that p21 is also involved in melanocyte differentiation (Jiang et al. 1994). Thus p21 plays a central role in a number of cellular processes that have in common the abrogation of cell proliferation, implicating this gene as being involved in cell cycle control (Fig. 4). These findings, together with the demonstration that p21 can inhibit cell growth of young dividing cells, suggest that p21 coding sequences may be useful for gene therapy aimed at inhibiting the growth of rapidly proliferating cells in some forms of cancer.

Although high level constitutive and stable expression of p21 is desirable for therapeutic use of this gene to prevent cell proliferation, such expression may also be efficient to prevent cell growth required for the in vitro isolation of stable expressor cell clones. Thus only cell clones that express p21 at a level below the threshold required for growth inhibition would be obtained. The ability to express p21 in an inducible fashion might circumvent this problem. This has been achieved again using the glucocorticoid regulated promoter of MMTV. A promoter conversion retroviral vector (Salmons et al. 1995; Saller et al. 1997) was constructed carrying p21 coding sequences that, after infection, expressed from the MMTV promoter (Fig. 5). The human bladder carcinoma-derived cell line, EJ (Parada et al. 1982), was infected with the promoter conversion vector carrying p21 and cell clones were isolated and analysed. These clones were shown to carry the p21 coding sequences under the transcriptional control of the MMTV promoter as expected (Mrochen et al. 1997). In the absence of dexamethasone, when p21 expression levels are low or even below the levels of detection, the cells grew well and 36% of the cells were found to be in the S phase of the cell cycle (EJ/p21; Table 1). However, addition of dexamethasone could be shown to stimulate p21 expression, and this was associated with a reduced growth potential with 27% of the cells in the S phase (EJ/p21; Table 1). This is a greater effect than that observed when

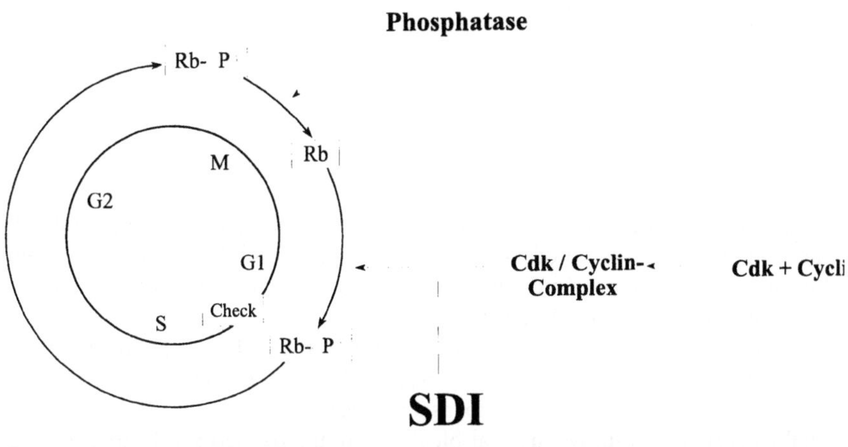

Fig. 4. The cell cycle and (senescent cell derived inhibitor) SDI. Expression of SDI inhibits the phosphorylation of the Rb protein by cyclin dependent kinase (Cdk)/cyclin complex during the G1 phase of the cell cycle. Lack of phosphorylated Rb during this period in the cell cycle results in arrest at the G1 checkpoint

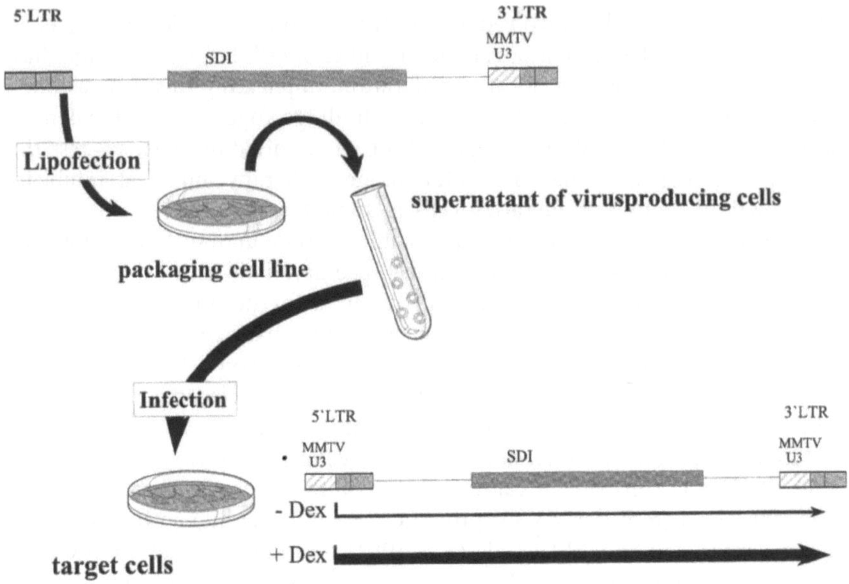

Fig. 5. ProCon vector carrying both the mouse mammary tumour virus (MMTV) promoter and the SDI therapeutic gene. Lipofection of packaging cells with a ProCon retroviral vector carrying the SDI gene gives rise to recombinant virions that can be used to infect target cells. After reverse transcription, the SDI gene is placed under the transcriptional control of the MMTV U3 region in the target cells. The glucocorticoid hormone inducibility of the MMTV U3 promoter allows expression of the SDI gene to be controlled in a dexamethasone dependent fashion

Table 1. Expression of senescent cell derived inhibitors reduces the number of dividing cells

Cells	% in S phase without dexamethasone	% in S phase with dexamethasone	Reduction
EJ	40.5	35.4	5.1
EJ/p21	35.7	27.0	8.7

non-genetically modified EJ cells are treated with dexamethasone (EJ; Table 1). Thus enhanced expression of p21 *in the same cell* can inhibit cell proliferation. The use of a strong constitutively active promoter should have more dramatic anti-proliferative therapeutic effect.

In addition to its potential use in cancer therapy, p21 may be an excellent therapeutic gene for the treatment of restenosis. This is a smooth muscle cell proliferative disorder of the cardiovascular system that results from conventional treatment to remove arterial blockage in atherosclerosis. Unfortunately, in 40% of patients, conventional treatment for atherosclerosis stimulates the growth of smooth muscle cells, leading to a secondary blockage (Nikol et al.

1996). Recently, it has been shown that p21 is normally involved in smooth muscle proliferation control and adenoviral vector mediated delivery of this protein can inhibit smooth muscle proliferation (Yang et al. 1996). However, it is known that adenoviral vectors cause inflammatory responses which may contribute to the development of restenosis in the long term. Retroviral vector mediated gene delivery may prove superior for the delivery of therapeutic genes like p21 for the treatment of restenosis.

Tumour Suppressor Genes

The tumour suppressor gene p53 is often mutated in a variety of cancers, particularly those with poor prognosis. Recently it has been shown, in a human clinical trial designed to treat lung cancer, that retroviral vector mediated delivery of p53 encoding sequences to cancer cells that no longer produce a functional p53 protein is beneficial (Roth et al. 1996). Even though maximally 20% of the cells in a given tumour had acquired the vector, tumour regression was still observed, presumably due to the transfer of p53 from genetically modified cells to non-modified cells, a phenomenon known as the bystander effect (Cai et al. 1993).

Suicide Genes

The use of genes encoding enzymes that convert non-toxic prodrugs to their active metabolites has been extensively studied in animal models of cancer and has met with mixed success in human clinical trials (Moolten 1994). These genes have been called "suicide genes" since they prime cells for death. The enzymes chosen are almost exclusively from non-mammalian organisms such as viruses or bacteria. The most commonly used gene is that encoding the thymidine kinase gene from herpes simplex virus, but some other examples are given in Table 2. An advantage to this kind of approach is that not all of the tumour cells (or implanted cells in the vicinity of the tumour) need to be ge-

Table 2. Some commonly used suicide genes and prodrugs

Gene	Source	Prodrug
Thymidine kinase	Herpes simplex virus	Ganciclovir Acyclovir
Thymidine kinase	Varicella zoster virus	Methoxypurine
Cytosine deaminase	*Escherichia coli*	5-Fluorocytosine
Guanine phosphoribosyl transferase	*Escherichia coli*	6-Thioxanthine
Cytochrome P450 2B1	Human, rodent	Cyclophosphamide Ifosfamide

netically modified since the active metabolites produced from the conversion of the prodrug are often diffusible, producing a bystander effect.

The mammalian cytochrome P450 family of enzymes are also of interest for cancer therapy. The cytochrome P450 2B1 gene is expressed in the liver and is important for classical cancer therapy regimes that utilize the chemotherapy agents cyclophosphamide and ifosfamide. These agents are usually given systemically, and only after cytochrome P450 2B1-mediated modification in the liver are the active toxic metabolites produced (Chang et al. 1993). The systemically distributed toxic metabolites cause alkylation of the DNA of cells. However, the effects of DNA alkylation are only seen during cell division, when such cells cannot replicate their DNA correctly and this results in cell death. Thus, in addition to the tumour cells, many different non-target cells, such as those of the haematopoietic system, are killed, resulting in severe side effects. The ability to relocate the site of conversion of the chemotherapeutic agent to the vicinity of the tumour itself would alleviate the side effects as well as increase the efficacy of the tumour specific cy-

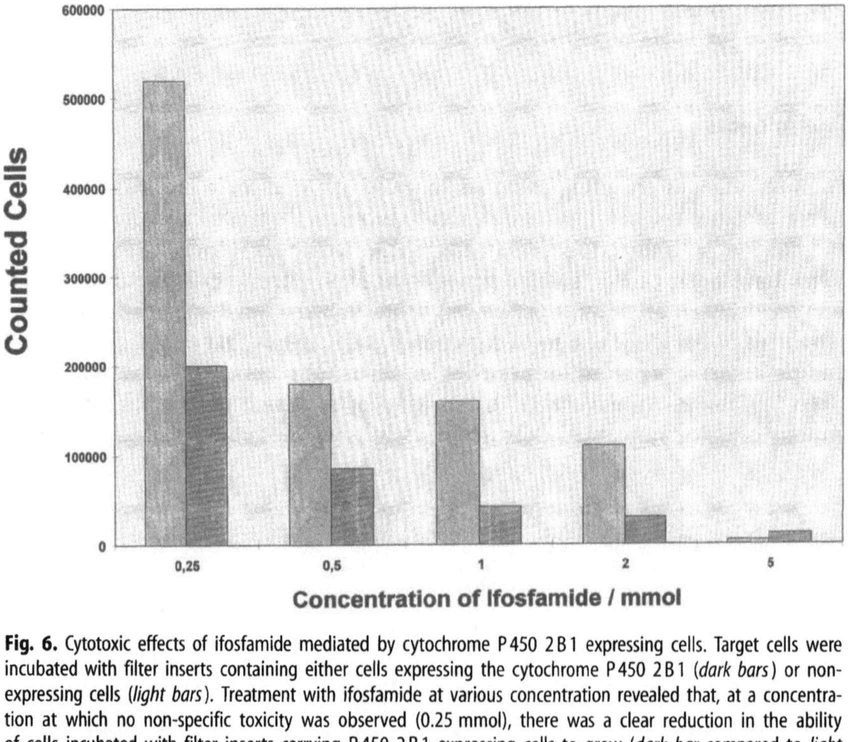

Fig. 6. Cytotoxic effects of ifosfamide mediated by cytochrome P450 2B1 expressing cells. Target cells were incubated with filter inserts containing either cells expressing the cytochrome P450 2B1 (*dark bars*) or non-expressing cells (*light bars*). Treatment with ifosfamide at various concentration revealed that, at a concentration at which no non-specific toxicity was observed (0.25 mmol), there was a clear reduction in the ability of cells incubated with filter inserts carrying P450 2B1 expressing cells to grow (*dark bar* compared to *light bar*). This difference was also clearly visible at higher concentrations, albeit with signs of non-specific toxicity (*light bars*). The data shown represent numbers of target cells counted after 5 days' exposure to ifosfamide corrected for non-specific growth effects of incubation with filter inserts containing P450 2B1 expressing or non-expressing cells

totoxicity. In a first step towards this goal, we have genetically modified cells in culture to express a rodent cytochrome P450 2B1 gene. Such cells become exquisitely sensitive to the cytotoxic effects of ifosfamide, since they are now able to convert this chemotherapeutic agent into its toxic metabolites whereas the parental, non-genetically modified cells are not. Further, this effect can be mediated to other cells as a result of the bystander effect (Fig. 6). This kind of approach has also been successful using genetically modified cells in animal model systems (Chen and Waxman 1995).

Conclusions and Perspectives

Gene therapy for the treatment of cancer as well as of monogenetic disorders, viral infections and cardiovascular disease holds much promise and many clinical trials are in progress. The judicious choice of therapeutic gene as well as of gene delivery system is important for the success of such approaches. The genes mentioned here are some of the most promising for the eventual treatment of cancer. The ability to target their delivery and limit their expression to tumour cells will contribute greatly both to safety and to efficacy.

References

Baum C, Hegewischbecker S, Eckert HG, Stocking C, Ostertag W (1995) Novel retroviral vectors for efficient expression of the multidrug-resistance (MDR-1) gene in early hematopoietic cells. J Virol 69:7541–7547

Cai DW, Mukhopadhyay T, Liu YJ, Fujiwara T, Roth JA (1993) Stable expression of the wild-type p53 gene in human lung cancer cells after retrovirus-mediated gene transfer. Hum Gene Ther 4:617–624

Chang TKH, Weber GF, Crespi CL, Waxman DJ (1993) Differential activation of cyclophosphamide and ifosphamide by cytochromes P450 2B and 3A in human liver microsomes. Cancer Res 53:5629–5637

Chen L, Waxman DJ (1995) Intratumoral activation and enhanced chemotherapeutic effect of oxazaphosphorines following cytochrome P-450 gene transfer: development of a combined chemotherapy/cancer gene therapy strategy. Cancer Res 55:581–589

Colombi MP, Forni G (1994) Cytokine gene transfer inhibition and tentative tumor therapy: where are we now? Immunol Today 15:48–51

Ewald D, Li M, Efrat S, Auer G, Wall RJ, Furth PA, Hennighausen L (1996) Time-sensitive reversal of hyperplasia in transgenic mice expressing SV40 T antigen. Science 273:1384–1386

Gu Y, Turck CW, Morgan DO (1993) Inhibition of CDK-2 activity in vivo by an associated 20K regulatory subunit. Nature 366:707–710

Günzburg WH, Salmons B (1992) Factors controlling the expression of mouse mammary tumour virus. Biochem J 283:625–632

Günzburg WH, Salmons B (1995) Virus vector design in gene therapy. Mol Med Today 1:410–417

Günzburg WH, Salmons B (1996) Gene transfer into mammalian cells: the road to human gene therapy. Gene Eng Biotechnol 16:81–98

Harper JW, Adami GR, Wei N, Keyomarsi K, Elledge SJ (1993) The p21 Cdk-interacting protein Cip1 is a potent inhibitor of G1 cyclin-dependent kinases. Cell 75:805–816

Herrmann F (1996) Clinical application of gene transfer. J Mol Med 74:213–221

Israel MA (1993) Molecular approaches to cancer therapy. Adv Cancer Res 61:57–85

Jiang H, Lin J, Su ZZ, Collart FR, Huberman E, Fisher PB (1994) Induction of differentiation in human promyelocytic HL-60 leukemia cells activates p21 WAF/CIP1, expression in the absence of p53. Oncogene 9:3397–3406

Johnson M, Dimitrov D, Vojta PJ, Barrett JC, Noda A, Pereira-Smith OM, Smith JR (1994) Evidence for a p53-independent pathway for upregulation of SDI1/CIP1/WAF1/p21 RNA in human cells. Mol Carcinog 11:59–64

Miller DG, Adam MA, Miller AD (1990) Gene transfer by retrovirus vectors occurs only in cells that are actively replicating at the time of infection. Mol Cell Biol 10:4139–4242

Moolten FL (1994) Drug sensitivity ("suicide") genes for selective cancer chemotherapy: use of suicide gene, e.g. herpes simplex virus thymidine-kinase, for prodrug activation and selective tumor killing. Cancer Gene Ther 1:279–287

Mrochen S, Klein D, Salmons B, Nikol S, Smith JR, Günzburg WH (1997) Inducible expression of p21SDI-1 from a promoter-conversion retroviral vector: a potential strategy for antiproliferative gene therapy. (submitted)

Nakanishi M, Adami GR, Robetorye RS, Noda A, Venable SF, Dimitrov D, Pereira-Smith O, Smith JR (1995) Exit from G_0 and entry into the cell cycle of cells expressing p21Sdil antisense RNA. Proc Natl Acad Sci USA 92:4352–4356

Nikol S, Huehns TY, Höfling B (1996) Molecular biology and post-angioplasty restenosis. Atherosclerosis 123:17–31

Noda A, Ning Y, Venable SF, Periera-Smith OM, Smith JR (1994) Cloning of senescent cell-derived inhibitors of DNA synthesis using an expression screen. Exp Cell Res 211:90–98

Parada LF, Tabin CJ, Shih C, Weinberg RA (1982) Human EJ bladder carcinoma oncogene is homologue of Harvey sarcoma virus ras gene. Nature 297:474–478

Rosenberg SA (1991) Immunotherapy and gene therapy of cancer. Cancer Res [Suppl] 51:5074–5079

Roth JA, Nguyen D, Lawrence DD, Kemp BL, Carrasco CH, Ferson DZ, Hong WK, Komani R, Lee J-J, Nesbitt JC, Pisters KMW, Putnam JB, Schea R, Shin DM, Walsh GL, Dolormente MM, Han C-I, Martin FD, Yen N, Xu K, Stephens LC, McDonnell TJ, Mukhopadhyay T, Cai D (1996) Retrovirus-mediated wild-type p53 gene transfer to tumors of patients with lung cancer. Nat Med 2:985–974

Saller RM, Özturk F, Salmons B, Günzburg WH (1997) Complete replacement of the U3 region in retroviral vectors with heterologous promoters for targeted expression. (submitted)

Salmons B, Erfle V, Brem G, Günzburg WH (1990) naf, a trans-regulating negative-acting factor encoded within the mouse mammary tumour virus open reading frame region. J Virol 64:6355–6359

Salmons B, Saller RM, Baumann J, Günzburg WH (1995) Construction of retroviral vectors for targeted delivery and expression of therapeutic genes. Leukemia 9 [Suppl 1]:53–60

Schiller JH, Storer BE, Witt PL, Alberti D, Tombes MB, Arzoomanian R, Proctor RA, McCarthy D, Brown RR, Voss SD, Remick SC, Grem JL, Borden EC, Trump DL (1991) Biological and clinical effects of intravenous tumor necrosis factor-alpha administered three times weekly. Cancer Res 51:1651–1658

Sparmann G, Walther W, Günzburg WH, Uckert W, Salmons B (1994) Conditional expression of human TFN-α: a system for inducible cytotoxicity. Int J Cancer 59:103–107

Xiong Y, Hannon GJ, Zhang H, Casso D, Kobayashi R, Beach D (1993) p21 is a universal inhibitor of cyclin kinases. Nature 366:701–704

Yang Z-Y, Simari RD, Perkins ND, San H, Gordon D, Nabel GJ, Nabel EG (1996) Role of the p21 cyclin-dependent kinase inhibitor in limiting intimal cell proliferation in response to arterial injury. Proc Natl Acad Sci USA 93:7905–7910

Specific *bcr-abl*-Directed Antisense Nucleic Acids and Ribozymes: A Tool for the Treatment of Chronic Myelogenous Leukemia?

R. Kronenwett[1] and R. Haas[1,2]

[1] Clinical Cooperation Unit Molecular Hematology/Oncology (460), German Cancer Research Center, Im Neuenheimer Feld 280, 69120 Heidelberg, Germany
[2] Department of Internal Medicine V, University of Heidelberg, Hospitalstrasse 3, 69115 Heidelberg, Germany

Introduction

Malignant diseases may result from abnormal gene expression either following pathological rearrangement, point mutations, overexpression of genes or integration of viral DNA. One method to switch off gene expression is the use of antisense nucleic acids, which hybridize to a part of the target RNA. The exact molecular mechanisms underlying the antisense effects are still not clear. The inhibition of protein expression is thought to result from steric hindrance of the antisense molecule after binding or from degradation of the mRNA by RNases as a consequence of hybridization (Fig. 1).

There are three different kinds of antisense nucleic acids (Table 1; Fig. 1). Antisense oligonucleotides are short sequences (<30 bases) of mostly deoxyribonucleotides which are synthesized chemically (Hélène and Toulmé 1990; Stein and Chang 1993). The stability of the oligonucleotides can be improved by chemical modifications such as phosphorothioate couplings along the deoxyribose backbones of the molecules. This type of short antisense oligonucleotides can be exogenously added to cells. Their delivery into cells can be enhanced by introducing chemical modifications such as cholesterol residues (Letsinger et al. 1989), by using cationic lipids as a transfection aid (Bennett et al. 1992; Capaccioli et al. 1993), or with the help of receptor-mediated uptake (Citro et al. 1992).

Another type of antisense nucleic acids are long-chain antisense RNAs, which must be endogenously expressed in cells by recombinant genes. Stable or transient introduction of antisense genes into cells can be achieved using nonviral or viral vectors such as retroviruses (Martiat et al. 1993; Junker et al. 1994; see also Fruehauf et al. and Günzburg et al., this volume), the adeno-associated virus type 2 (Ponnazhagan et al. 1994; see also Ogniben and Haas, this volume), or eukaryotic expression plasmids (Sczakiel and Pawlita 1991). A third group of RNA-targeting molecules are ribozymes. Ribozymes are catalytic RNAs which bind their target by antisense arms and cleave at a specific consensus sequence (Marshall et al. 1994; James and Al-Shamkhani

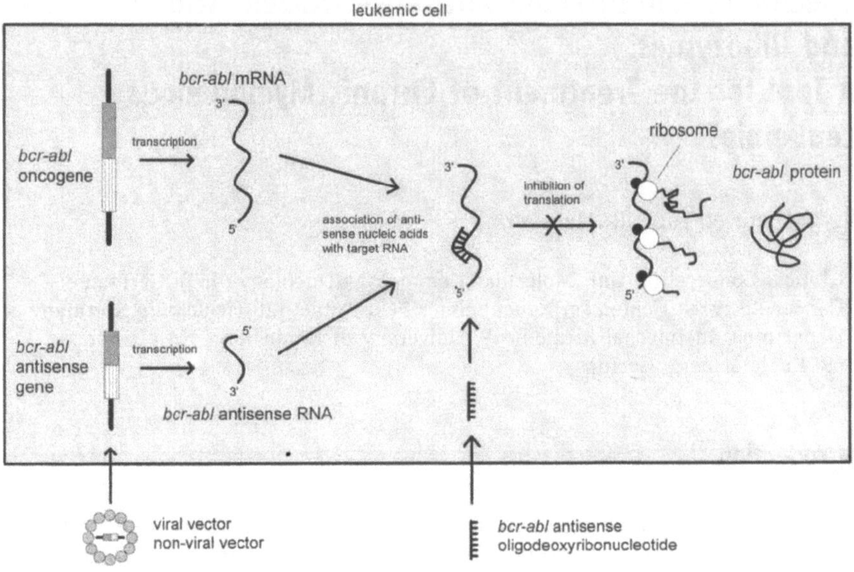

Fig. 1. Delivery of antisense nucleic acids into leukemic cells and effect on oncogene expression

Table 1. Types and delivery of antisense nucleic acids and ribozymes

Antisense nucleic acid	Delivery to living cells
Antisense DNA (oligodeoxyribonucleotides)	Exogenous application Improvement of cellular uptake and prevention of degradation by chemical modifications
Antisense RNA	Recombinant antisense genes Viral and nonviral vectors
Ribozymes (antisense RNA+RNA-cleaving domain)	Recombinant genes Exogenous application of chemically synthesized ribozymes

1995; see also James, this volume). The functional combination of binding and cleavage in one molecule makes them independent from cellular RNases. Like antisense oligodeoxyribonucleotides, ribozymes can be synthesized chemically and delivered to cells exogenously. Alternatively, they may be introduced into cells by recombinant genes for continuous expression of catalytic RNA.

The antisense methodology provides a therapeutic modality for patients with malignancies caused by or associated with a tumor-specific abnormality of gene expression. The targeting of genes that are involved in the malignant phenotype but not expressed in normal cells may selectively eliminate neoplastic cells. Chronic myelogenous leukemia (CML) is such a disease, with a cytogenetic abnormality present in 90%–95% of patients. The hallmark is the Philadelphia chromosome, which results from a reciprocal chromosomal translocation between chromosome 9 and 22 (for review see Kurzrock et al. 1988). The *bcr-abl* fusion gene consists of *bcr* sequences from chromosome 22 at its 5′ portion and *abl* sequences from chromosome 9 at the 3′ portion. The *bcr-abl* gene encodes for a 210-kDa protein which is thought to play a pivotal role in the pathogenesis of CML. This view is supported by studies in mice where the expression of the *bcr-abl* gene causes lymphohematopoietic malignancies resembling CML (Daley et al. 1990; Kelliher et al. 1990). The chromosomal breakpoints span defined regions within the *bcr* and *abl* genes. Following splicing of the *bcr-abl* transcript, there are in most cases of CML two alternative types of messenger RNA, referred to as b3a2 and b2a2. Compared to the b2a2 RNA, the b3a2 RNA contains the additional exon *bcr* 3. In consequence, there are two fusion points constituting potential target sequences for antisense nucleic acids.

Selectivity of *bcr-abl*-Directed Antisense Nucleic Acids

There are many reports on the inhibition of Philadelphia-chromosome-positive (Ph+) leukemic cells by antisense nucleic acids or ribozymes directed to the *bcr-abl* fusion sequences. The results were heterogenous and even contradictory in some instances (Nichols 1995). Specific inhibition, nonspecific inhibition, and no inhibition of proliferation of leukemic cells were described. Problems still exist concerning the choice of target region, the lack of appropriate controls, and the suitability of model cells. Another question relates to the sequence specificity for the *bcr-abl* target RNA, which differs only slightly from nontarget sequences. The degree of overlap of the antisense sequences with wild-type *bcr* and *abl* could result in adverse side effects in normal cells. The functions of *bcr* and *abl* are still not known but they are apparently involved in cell cycle control and signal transduction (Sawyers et al. 1994; Voncken et al. 1995). Therefore, antisense inhibitors should efficiently bind to the *bcr-abl* fusion sequence but only poorly to the wild-type sequences *bcr* and *abl*.

The sequence selectivity of short-chain antisense oligonucleotides can be examined in vitro by the melting temperatures of the resulting double strands: where there are nonmatching nucleotides within an antisense oligonucleotide the melting temperature decreases and the duplex becomes less stable. The case is different with long stretches of complementary sequences (>30–40 nucleotides), where discrimination between a completely matching target and a sequence that differs in only a few bases is not possible on the basis of melting temperature. Still, for long-chain antisense RNA the rate of association of complementary sequences in vitro correlates with the efficacy in vivo, while the stability of the antisense RNA/target RNA duplex does not. In order to identify *bcr-abl*-specific antisense inhibitors we looked for antisense sequences which bind rapidly to the fusion RNA but poorly to either of the two wild-type sequences *bcr* and *abl*. For this purpose the association kinetics of complementary nucleic acids were examined.

Identification of Selectively Binding Complementary RNA

For identification of fast-hybridizing antisense species out of a pool of successively 3′ shortened *bcr-abl*-directed antisense RNAs an in vitro selection method was used as described by Rittner et al. (1993) and Kronenwett and Sczakiel (1997) (Fig. 2). From a parental *bcr-abl* fusion point b3a2 spanning

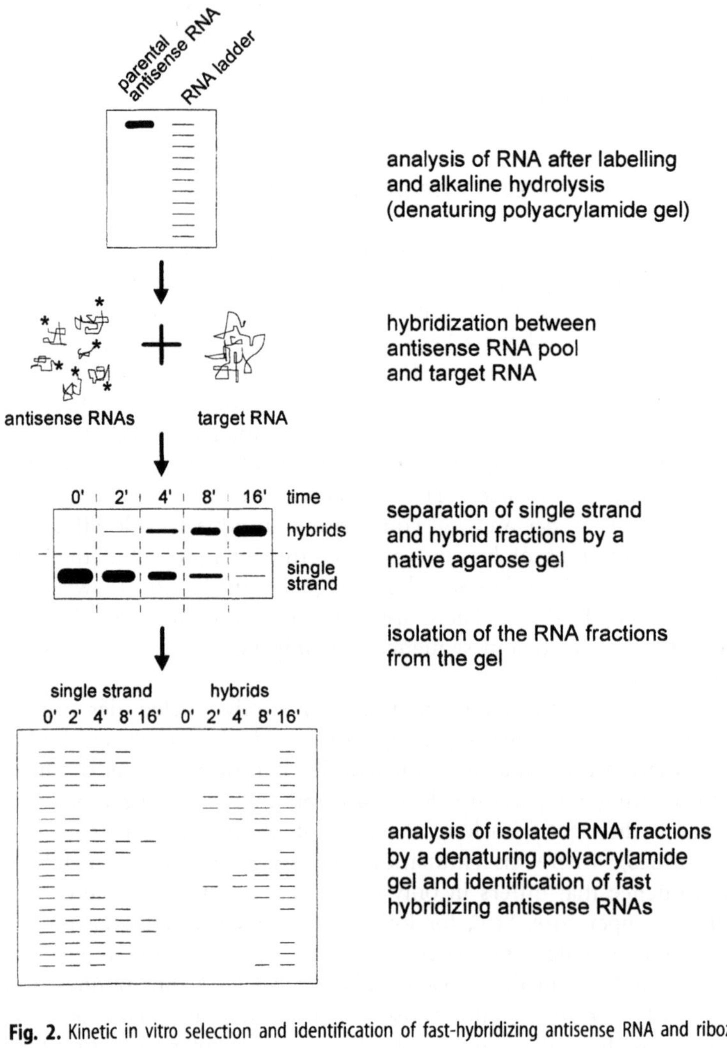

Fig. 2. Kinetic in vitro selection and identification of fast-hybridizing antisense RNA and ribozyme species

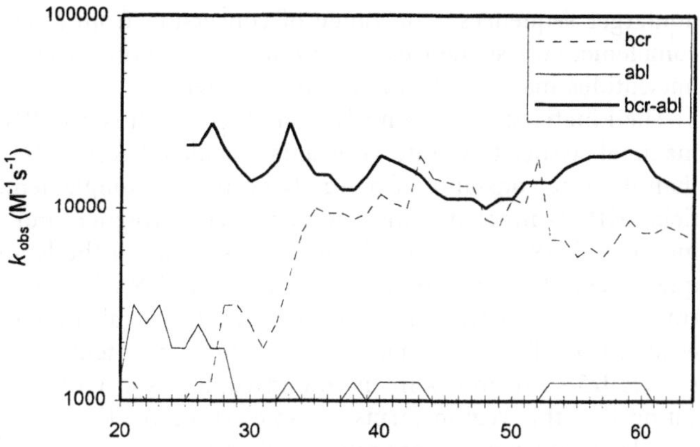

Fig. 3. Association rate constants (k_{obs}) for annealing with *bcr-abl, abl* and *bcr* target RNA as a function of chain length of the antisense strands. For calculating association rate constants annealing reactions were analyzed as described in Fig. 2, and band intensities on the polyacrylamide gel were quantified using a PhosphorImager

antisense RNA a pool of RNA species was generated by alkaline hydrolysis. The RNA species had a radioactively labeled 5′ end in common and differed by the length of the 3′ portion. For each individual antisense species the annealing rates with *bcr-abl, abl* and *bcr* target RNA, respectively, were measured. The association rate constants of antisense RNA species derived from a 79mer parental antisense RNA with 50 nucleotides complementary to the *bcr* portion and 12 nucleotides complementary to the *abl* sequences of the *bcr-abl* transcript are shown in Fig. 3. Out of a pool of antisense RNA species successively shortened at the anti-*bcr* portion, oligomeric sequences of between 25 and 31 nucleotides were identified which anneal at least ten-fold faster with the *bcr-abl* RNA than with either of the wild-type transcripts *bcr* or *abl.* Longer antisense RNA species of between 34 and 39 nucleotides as well as between 53 and 62 nucleotides also showed kinetically selective annealing (Kronenwett et al. 1996).

The in vitro assay for identifying fast-annealing antisense species was performed with RNA. To demonstrate that the findings are also true for DNA oligonucleotides, which are often used in cell culture experiments, annealing reactions between antisense deoxyribonucleotides and target RNA were examined by adding RNaseH. RNaseH recognizes RNA-DNA hybrids and cleaves the RNA portion. In the presence of selected oligodeoxyribonucleotide sequences and RNaseH the *bcr-abl* transcript was specifically hydrolyzed out of a mixture containing *abl* and *bcr* sequences as well, indicating that selectivity is independent of the type of nucleic acid used (Kronenwett et al. 1996).

Our study demonstrates the possibility of identifying specific antisense inhibitors directed against particular sequences which differ only slightly from nontarget sequences. The range of conversion from selective to nonselective complementary sequences is very small, as addition or deletion of only few nucleotides may result in a loss of selectivity.

The kinetic studies using *bcr-abl*-directed antisense RNAs showed that the maximal association rate constants calculated were 10- to 100-fold smaller than the rate constants of naturally occurring complementary RNAs and artificial HIV-1-directed antisense sequences (Wagner and Simons 1994; Homann et al. 1993). The low kinetic accessibility of the *bcr-abl* b3a2 fusion sequence could be explained by a stable local RNA structure. The extent of intramolecular interactions is reflected by the local folding potential (Sczakiel et al. 1993). The computer-calculated folding potential in the vicinity of the *bcr-abl* b3a2 fusion point is low in comparison with other sequences, indicating that this region forms a stable structure (Kronenwett et al. 1996). The *bcr-abl* fusion point sequences are therefore not easily accessible to complementary nucleic acids, and further structural investigations of the *bcr-abl* RNA are necessary for development of improved antisense inhibitors.

Development of Specific *bcr-abl*-Directed Ribozymes

Ribozymes are RNA molecules which bind their target by complementary sequences and cleave them at a specific recognition motif. Therefore, the biological efficacy of ribozymes in cells depends on fast association with the target RNA. For identification of potent ribozyme inhibitors kinetic studies are required, as in the case of antisense RNA. It is known for hammerhead ribozymes that one of the two antisense arms can be deleted, giving rise to an asymmetric molecule with full cleavage activity (Tabler et al. 1994). We designed asymmetric hammerhead ribozymes which bind the *bcr-abl* RNA by one antisense arm. Binding and cleavage occur on opposite sides of the fusion point (Fig. 4).

The asymmetric design provides two advantages:

(1) association kinetics can be performed with ribozymes successively shortened at the antisense arm for the identification of fast and selectively hybridizing ribozyme species;
(2) selectivity for the *bcr-abl* fusion transcript can be improved, because only if the match is perfect will the target RNA be cleaved.

Selective cleavage of the *bcr-abl* RNA by an in vitro selected, fast hybridizing asymmetric hammerhead ribozyme was demonstrated under experimental conditions in which both the association and the cleavage step contribute to specific destruction of the target (Kronenwett et al. 1996). Using a selected ribozyme the half life of the *bcr-abl* RNA was in the range between 10 and 12 h (Fig. 4, lower part). Neither *bcr* nor *abl* RNA was cleaved by the *bcr-abl*-directed ribozyme. Another possibility for achieving selectivity for the *bcr-abl* RNA are ribozymes which are connected with an antisense arm by anchor sequences (Pachuk et al. 1994). These data demonstrate that chimeric

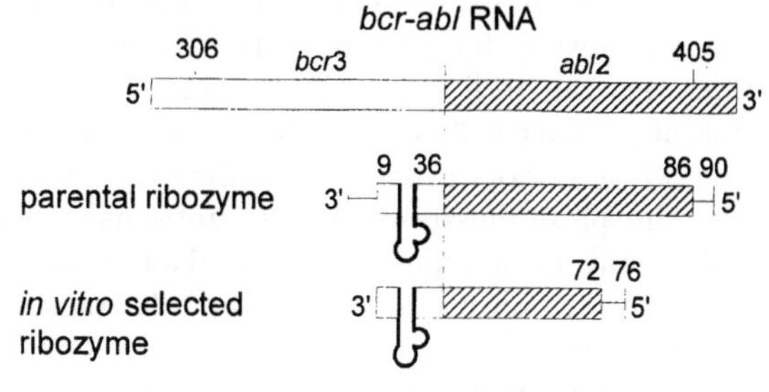

Ribozyme	Temperature (°C)	Half-life (hours)		
		bcr-abl	*abl*1b	*bcr*
in vitro selected ribozyme	37	9.6	>150	>150
		11.6	>150	>150

Fig. 4. Design and in vitro cleavage activity under single turnover conditions of a *bcr-abl*-directed hammerhead ribozyme

fusion transcripts are selectively cleaved by ribozymes using special constructions of the catalytic RNAs.

Efficacy of *bcr-abl*-Directed Antisense Oligonucleotides in Cell Culture and CML SCID Mouse Models

To test whether the oligomeric nucleic acid sequences that we identified by kinetic in vitro selection can specifically affect the proliferation of t(9;22)-positive cells, the *bcr-abl*-positive cell line K562 and primary cells from patients with de novo CML were treated with phosphorothioate antisense oligodeoxyribonucleotides (23mer and 28mer). In a series of three experiments neither the proliferation of K562 cells in suspension culture nor the colony-forming ability of primary cells in semisolid culture assays was affected. We assume that the poor cellular uptake of the molecules as demonstrated using radioactively labeled oligonucleotides accounts for the lack of efficacy. Our efforts are therefore concentrated on methods to improve delivery of oligonucleotides into cells.

Our results are consistent with the heterogeneous and contradictory reports about inhibition of Ph+ cells by antisense oligonucleotides published in the last few years. Most of the studies were performed using CML cell lines (Skorski et al. 1994; Smetsers et al. 1994), although immortalized cell lines are different from primary cells of patients with CML. For example, the cell line K562 has many chromosomal aberrations and contains multiple *bcr-*

abl alleles (Collins and Groudine 1983). Immortalized cell lines are therefore not appropriate for use in evaluating the efficacy of antisense oligonucleotides. Several studies were performed using clonogenic assays for the cultivation of primary cells from patients in chronic phase or in blastic transformation. Most authors observed specific or nonspecific effects of phosphodiester- or phosphorothioate-modified antisense deoxyribonucleotides (Nichols 1995). Still, most reports lack any data on the influence of the antisense oligonucleotides on the amount of *bcr-abl* transcripts or the level of p210 protein expression. This kind of assessment could provide the evidence to demonstrate a target-specific antisense effect. Another open question relates to the phase of CML most suitable for antisense treatment (Vaerman et al. 1993).

For evaluating the in vivo efficacy of antisense oligonucleotides a severe combined immunodeficient (SCID) mouse model was used (Skorski et al. 1994). SCID mice were injected with Ph+ BV173 cells and systemically treated for 9 days with a *bcr-abl*-directed phosphorothioate-modified 26mer antisense oligodeoxyribonucleotide. The treated mice survived 10 weeks longer than the mice in the control group. These experiments suggest that in vivo approaches in CML patients may be effective.

Alternative Target Sequences

Although the *bcr-abl* mRNA is a specific target for CML cells, other target sequences are also worth examining. It is conceivable that after treatment with *bcr-abl*-directed antisense oligonucleotides a significant number of leukemic cells survive due to lack of *bcr-abl* RNA expression. Using a combination of antisense oligonucleotides directed against different targets may exert an additive effect to circumvent resistance. A potential target site in Ph+ cells is the proto-oncogene c-*myb*, which encodes for a DNA-binding transcription factor (Lyon et al. 1994). It is differentially expressed in leukemic cells compared with normal cells, and it was shown that a c-*myb*-directed antisense oligonucleotide could inhibit clonogenic growth of primary cells of patients in blastic transformation, but had little effect on normal hematopoietic progenitor cells (Calabretta et al. 1991). Studies on SCID mice transplanted with the cell line K562 resulted in prolonged survival of animals treated with c-*myb* antisense oligomers in comparison with controls (Ratajczak et al. 1992).

Since c-*myb*-directed antisense oligonucleotides can inhibit normal progenitor cell growth to some extent (Gewirtz and Calabretta 1988), a limitation could be that, as in the case of chemotherapy, the effect is due to differential inhibition of normal versus leukemic cell proliferation and that the benefit of selectivity is lost.

Potential Clinical Application of Antisense Nucleic Acids and Ribozymes in Patients with CML

The possibilities of the clinical use of synthetic antisense oligonucleotides and ribozymes in patients with CML include ex vivo treatment of cells and systemic in vivo administration.

Normal, Ph–, nonclonal hematopoietic progenitor cells with suppression of later stages of normal hematopoiesis are maintained in CML patients (Coulombel et al. 1983). Therefore, normal hematopoietic progenitor cells can be harvested from bone marrow for autologous transplantation after high-dose cytotoxic therapy (Santos 1990). Normal Ph– peripheral blood stem cells were collected during the early period of marrow recovery following G-CSF-supported cytotoxic chemotherapy from patients with CML in chronic phase (Carella et al. 1993; see also Mahon et al., this volume). Since genetic marker studies showed that Ph+ cells in autologous transplants of patients with CML contribute to relapse (Deisseroth et al. 1994; see also Brenner, this volume), it might be beneficial to remove residual leukemic cells from autografts using ex vivo purging such as treatment with oncogene-directed antisense nucleic acids alone or in combination with conventional purging agents. A pilot study for ex vivo purging of CD34+-enriched bone marrow from patients with CML in chronic and accelerated phase using c-*myb*-directed antisense oligonucleotides has been initiated at the University of Pennsylvania in Philadelphia (Gewirtz et al. 1996; Calabretta et al. 1996). For purging, CD34+ bone marrow cells are treated for 24 h at 37 °C with phosphorothioate-modified oligonucleotides. After myeloablative therapy the purged marrow is reinfused into the patient. So far, in four of five evaluable patients in chronic phase 85%–100% Ph– metaphases were detected 3 months after engraftment. One patient treated more than 2 years ago has 80% normal metaphases.

The second possibility in the therapeutic application of antisense oligomers is systemic treatment. Supported by the efficacy in the CML SCID mouse model (Ratajczak et al. 1992), a phase-I dose escalation trial of systemically applied phosphorothioate-modified c-*myb* antisense oligodeoxyribonucleotides in patients with CML in blast crisis and patients with refractory acute leukemia was started in Philadelphia (Gewirtz et al. 1996; Calabretta et al. 1996). The antisense oligomers were administered by continuous intravenous infusion over a period of 7 days in a 28-day repeating cycle at dose levels ranging between 0.3 and 2 mg/kg per day. So far, no drug-related toxicities have been observed, but the therapeutic benefit is still unclear.

Conclusions

The question whether specific *bcr-abl*-directed antisense inhibitors provide an effective alternative or additional therapeutic approach for the treatment of CML cannot yet be answered. In regard to the problem of selectivity in antisense experiments, our studies demonstrate that complementary sequences hybridizing specifically with the *bcr-abl* target RNA and sparing the wild-type transcripts *bcr* and *abl* can be identified. Whether these specific antisense molecules are effective in cell cultures or following in vivo administration to patients awaits further studies. To improve the potential biological effects of antisense nucleic acids and ribozymes, new oligonucleotide chemistries and better methods of delivery to cells are needed to increase cellular uptake, intracellular transport, and the stability of the therapeutic molecules. Future studies should focus on structural investigations of the *bcr-abl* RNA in order to improve the interaction between the antisense inhibitor and the target transcript. It should also be taken into account that inactivation of the *bcr-abl* oncogene may possibly not be sufficient for inhibition of CML cells, and that other target sequences must be identified. Clinical studies are needed to evaluate more effective schedules of administration of antisense or ribozyme inhibitors, alone or in combination with conventional cytotoxic drugs. Despite these unanswered questions, the antisense strategy is a promising disease-specific antineoplastic treatment modality.

Acknowledgments. We wish to thank G. Sczakiel, M. Deichmann, M. Kirsch, and U. Steidl for their valuable comments and discussion as well as their expert technical support.

References

Bennett CF, Chiang M-Y, Chan H, Shoemaker JEE, Mirabelli CK (1992) Cationic lipids enhance cellular uptake and activity of phosphorothioate antisense oligonucleotides. Mol Pharmacol 41:1023–1033

Calabretta B, Sims RR, Valtieri M, Caracciolo D, Szczylik C, Venturelli D, Ratajczak MZ, Beran M, Gewirtz AM (1991) Normal and leucemic cells manifest differential sensitivity to inhibitory effects of c-myb antisense oligodeoxynucleotides: an in vitro study relevant to bone marrow purging. Proc Natl Acad Sci USA 88:2351–2355

Calabretta B, Skorski T, Ratajczak MZ, Gewirtz AM (1996) Antisense strategies in the treatment of leukemias. Semin Oncol 23:78–87

Capaccioli S, Di Pasquale G, Mini E, Mazzei T, Quattrone A (1993) Cationic lipids improve antisense oligonucleotide uptake and prevent degradation in cultured cells and in human serum. Biochem Biophys Res Commun 197:818–825

Carella AM, Podestà M, Frassoni F et al. (1993) Collection of 'normal' blood repopulating cells during early hemopoietic recovery after intensive conventional chemotherapy in chronic myelogenous leukemia. Bone Marrow Transplant 12:267–271

Citro G, Perrotti D, Cucco C, D'Agnano I, Sacchi A, Zupi G, Calabretta B (1992) Inhibition of leukemia cell proliferation by receptor-mediated uptake of c-myb antisense oligodeoxynucleotides. Proc Natl Acad Sci USA 89:7031–7035

Collins SJ, Groudine MT (1983) Rearrangement and amplification of c-abl sequences in the human chronic myelogenous leukemia cell line K-562. Proc Natl Acad Sci USA 80:4813–4817

Coulombel L, Kalousek DK, Eaves CJ, Gupta CM, Eaves AC (1983) Long-term bone marrow culture reveals chromosomally normal hematopoietic progenitor cells in patients with Ph chromosome positive chronic myelogenous leukemia. N Engl J Med 308:1493–1498

Daley GQ, Van Etten RA, Baltimore D (1990) Induction of chronic myelogenous leukemia in mice by the P210 bcr/abl gene of the Philadelphia chromosome. Science 247:824–830

Deisseroth AB, Zu Z, Claxton D et al (1994) Genetic marking shows that Ph+ cells present in autologous transplants of chronic myelogenous leukemia (CML) contribute to relapse after autologous bone marrow transplantation in CML. Blood 83:3068–3076
Gewirtz AM, Calabretta B (1988) A c-myb antisense oligodeoxynucleotide inhibits normal human hematopoiesis in vitro. Science 242:1303–1306
Gewirtz AW, Luger S, Sokol D, Gowdin B, Stadtmauer E, Reccio A, Ratajczak MZ (1996) Treating human myelogenous leukemia with c-myb antisense oligonucleotides: two years clinical experience. J Invest Med 44:279a
Hélène C, Toulmé JJ (1990) Specific regulation of gene expression by antisense, sense and antigene nucleic acids. Biochim Biophys Acta 1049:99–125
Homann M, Rittner K, Sczakiel G (1993) Complementary large loops determine the rate of duplex formation in vitro in case of an effective antisense RNA directed against the human immunodeficiency virus type 1. J Mol Biol 233:7–15
James W, Al-Shamkhani A (1995) RNA enzymes as tools for gene ablation. Curr Opin Biotechnol 6:44–49
Junker U, Rittner K, Hohmann M, Bevec D, Böhnlein E, Sczakiel G (1994) Reduction in replication of the human T cell lines by polymerase III-driven transcription of chimeric tRNA-antisense RNA genes. Antisense Res Dev 4:165–172
Kelliher MA, McLaughlin J, Witte ON, Rosenberg N (1990) Induction of a chronic myelogenous leukemia-like syndrome in mice with v-abl and BCR/ABL. Proc Natl Acad Sci USA 87:6649–6653
Kronenwett R, Haas R, Sczakiel G (1996) Kinetic selectivity of complementary nucleic acids: bcr-abl-directed antisense RNA and ribozymes. J Mol Biol 259:632–644
Kronenwett R, Sczakiel G (1997) Selection of fast-hybridizing complementary RNA species in vitro. In: Turner PC (ed) Ribozyme protocols. Methods in molecular biology, vol. 74. Humana, Totowa, pp 281–288
Kurzrock R, Gutterman JU, Talpaz M (1988) The molecular genetics of Philadelphia chromosome-positive leukemias. N Engl J Med 319:990–998
Letsinger RL, Zhang G, Sun DK, Ikeuchi T, Sarin PS (1989) Cholesteryl-conjugated oligonucleotides: synthesis, properties, and activity as inhibitors of replication of human immunodeficiency virus in cell culture. Proc Natl Acad Sci USA 86:6553–6556
Lyon J, Robinson C, Watson R (1994) The role of myb proteins in normal and neoplastic cell proliferation. Crit Rev Oncog 5:373–388
Marshall P, Thompson JB, Eckstein F (1994) Inhibition of gene expression with ribozymes. Cell Mol Neurobiol 14:5523–5538
Martiat P, Lewalle P, Taj A, Philippe M, Larondelle Y, Vaerman JL, Wildmann C, Goldman JM, Michaux JL (1993) Retroviral transduced antisense sequences stably suppress p210 brc-abl expression and inhibit the proliferation of bcr-abl-containing cell lines. Blood 81:502–509
Nichols GL (1995) Antisense oligonucleotides as therapeutic agents for chronic myelogenous leukemia. Antisense Res Dev 5:67–69
Pachuk CJ, Yoon K, Moelling K, Coney LR (1994) Selective cleavage of bcr-abl chimeric RNAs by a ribozyme targeted to non-continuous sequences. Nucleic Acids Res 22:301–307
Ponnazhagan S, Nallari ML, Srivastava A (1994) Suppression of human α-blobin gene expression mediated by the recombinant adeno-associated virus 2-based antisense vectors. J Exp Med 179:733–738
Ratajczak MZ, Kant JA, Luger SM, Huiya N, Zhang J, Zon G, Gewirtz AM (1992) In vivo treatment of human leukemia in a SCID mouse model with c-myb antisense oligonucleotides. Proc Natl Acad Sci USA 89:11823–11827
Rittner K, Burmester C, Sczakiel G (1993) In vitro selection of fast-hybridizing and effective antisense RNAs directed against the human immunodeficiency virus type 1. Nucleic Acids Res 21:1381–1387
Santos GW (1990) Bone marrow transplantation in hematologic malignancies: current status. Cancer 65:786–791
Sawyers CL, McLaughlin J, Goga A, Havlik M, Witte ON (1994) The nuclear tyrosine kinase c-abl negatively regulates cell growth. Cell 77:121–131

Sczakiel G, Pawlita M (1991) Inhibition of human immunodeficiency virus type 1 replication in human T cells stably expressing antisense RNA. J Virol 65:468–472

Sczakiel G, Homann M, Rittner K (1993) Computer-acided search for effective antisense RNA target sequences of the human immunodeficiency virus type 1. Antisense Res Dev 3:45–52

Skorski T, Nieborowska-Skorska M, Nicolaides NC, Szczylik C, Iversen P, Iozzo RV, Zon G, Calabretta B (1994) Suppression of Philadelphia[1] leukemia cell growth in mice by BCR/ABL antisense oligodeoxynucleotide. Proc Natl Acad Sci USA 91:4504–4508

Smetsers TFCM, Skorski T, van de Locht LTF, Wessels HMC, Pennings AHM, de Witte T, Calabretta B, Mensink EJBM (1994) Antisense BCR-ABL oligonucleotides induce apoptosis in the Philadelphia chromosome-positive cell line BV 173. Leukemia 8:129–140

Stein CA, Chang YC (1993) Antisense oligonucleotides as therapeutic agents – is the bullet really magical? Science 261:1004–1012

Tabler M, Homann M, Tzortzakaki S, Sczakiel G (1994) A three nucleotide helix I is sufficient for full activity of a hammerhead ribozyme: advantages of an asymmetric design. Nucleic Acids Res 22:3958–3965

Vaerman JL, Lewalle P, Martiat P (1993) Antisense inhibition of P210 bcr-abl in chronic myeloid leukemia. Stem Cells 11 Suppl 3:89–95

Voncken JW, van Schaick H, Kaartinen V, Deemer K, Coates T, Landing B, Pattengale P, Dorseuil O, Bokoch GM, Groffen J, Heisterkamp N (1995) Increased neutrophil respiratory burst in *bcr*-null mutants. Cell 80:719–728

Wagner EGH, Simons RW (1994) Antisense RNA control in bacteria, phage and plasmids. Annu Rev Microbiol 48:713–740

The Use of Ribozymes in Gene Therapy Approaches to AIDS

W. James

Sir William Dunn School of Pathology, University of Oxford, Oxford, OX1 3RE, UK

Introduction

The development of effective therapies or promising vaccines for AIDS has been a goal of international research for more than a decade but the mutability of the virus and complex pathogenesis of the disease have made these goals extremely elusive. Only recently have traditional chemotherapeutic approaches begun to look promising. As an alternative, a number of groups have been investigating the potential of antiviral RNAs expressed from recombinant viral vectors to form the basis of a gene therapy for the disease. In this paper, I outline several challenges to the efficient deployment of a gene therapy for AIDS, particularly the efficient transduction of heamopoietic cells and their engraftment in a physiologically competent form, and review the current approaches designed to overcome them.

Gene Therapy

Gene therapy approaches to disease can be divided conceptually into a variety of distinct techniques. The majority of inherited disorders result from point mutations in particular genes, for example, the commoner forms of haemophilia, cystic fibrosis, muscular dystrophy and the thalassaemias. For these diseases, the approach being taken is often termed "gene replacement therapy", in which a copy of the wild-type allele of the gene in question is inserted into the genome of a genetic vector, which is then introduced into the appropriate tissue of the patient in order for the normal form of the protein to be expressed. This approach should, perhaps, be called "gene augmentation therapy", as the mutant allele remains in situ. The challenges to these approaches to therapy are numerous. For example, the target tissue and its stem cells are often poorly accessible or non-proliferative, the vector or delivery system is frequently inefficient or causes undue side effects, and it may often be difficult to obtain appropriately regulated, long-term expression of the recombinant gene in vivo. A problem of a more fundamental kind emerges when the diseases is not fully recessive or when exact levels of gene expression are required. This might be a problem in, for example, the thalassaemias and several of the genetic disease of the eye. In principle, the ideal approach would be gene conversion therapy, in which the sequence of the mutant allele were reverted in situ to that of the wild-type allele. Recent papers from the group of Kmiec claim success in developing a method for gene conversion (Cole-Strauss et al. 1996; Yoon et al. 1996) but the generalizability and reproducibility of their methodology is open to question. Finally, those diseases that result from the expression of a dominant, mutant allele, the inappropriate expression of a wild-type allele or the expression of foreign genes, might be amenable to gene inhibition therapy, in which a gene whose product interferes with the expression of the unwanted gene product is introduced into the target cells.

Antisense RNA and HIV Infection

It is this last category of gene therapy approach that may be applicable in AIDS. AIDS can be thought of, simplistically, as an acquired, dominant genetic disease, in that without the expression of the foreign viral genes within the T helper lymphocytes, macrophages and related cells, the disease would not be manifested. An approach to gene inhibition therapy for AIDS has involved the use of retroviral or other vectors to introduce messenger-complementary, or antisense, RNA-encoding genes into HIV-susceptible cells (Rhodes and James 1990; Sczakiel et al. 1990). It was found that these were reasonably effective methods for inhibiting the replication of HIV in cell culture, although the effects were somewhat transitory. Effective antisense RNAs were found to be at least approximately 50 nt long and be characterized by a lower-than-average degree of intramolecular base pairing (Rhodes and James 1991).

Ribozymes

With the discovery that catalytic RNAs, ribozymes, could be manipulated to produce RNA molecules that cleaved target RNAs of choice (Hampel and Tritz 1989; Haseloff and Gerlach 1988; Uhlenbeck 1987), it became apparent that one could endow the antisense RNA with additional inhibitory effect by including a ribozyme motiv. Of the several types of ribozyme now available, the hammerhead has the greatest flexibility of target site (Perriman et al. 1992) and methods have been designed to transform almost any antisense RNA-encoding gene into a catalytic antisense gene (Tabler and Tsagris 1991). These methods were exploited rapidly to demonstrate the ability of recombinant ribozymes to inhibit HIV expression in transduced cells in culture (Sarver et al. 1990; Chen et al. 1992; Dropulic et al. 1992; Lo et al. 1992; Ojwang et al. 1992; Crisell et al. 1993; Homann et al. 1993; Yu et al. 1993). However, the examples of inhibitory ribozymes that appear in press do not fully represent the true picture: most ribozymes are non-inhibitory.

What makes a ribozyme inhibitory?

A lively debate has opened up to address this question. On the one hand, the standard kinetic framework, derived from cell-free assays (Hertel et al. 1994), leads one towards the development of ribozymes whose efficiency, as indicated by the ratio between Km and k_{cat}, is maximal. It was soon discovered that ribozymes with very short flanking antisense arms (6–8 nt) were more catalytic than those with longer arms (Fedor and Uhlenbeck 1990; Goodchild and Kohli 1991). A number of factors played a part in this. First, if the assays are done under standard enzyme conditions, in which there is substantially more substrate than ribozyme, then only those ribozymes that can dissociate from their cleaved products will have a true k_{cat}. Consequently, the dissociation step, which is not available to ribozymes with long antisense arms, drives ribozyme design towards the short-arm paradigm. However, under physiologically relevant conditions, in which long substrate mRNAs can take up a range of complex secondary structures, and particularly – as is normal using genetic vectors – if the ribozyme is itself embedded in a long RNA of non-complementary sequence, the binding step between the ribozyme and its target is rate-limiting (Bertrand et al. 1994). A number of studies have shown that ribozymes with longer antisense arms are often more effective in cells than those with short ones (Crisell et al. 1993; Tabler et al. 1994), and this may reflect the rarity of suitable sites for the nucleation of hybridization between two long, complementary RNAs. For a particular family of ribozymes, we have recently shown that the role of long antisense arms is to entrap those rare regions of the target RNA that are favourable for hybridization (S. Thompson et al., unpublished). These favourable target regions and suitable ribozyme constructs can be successfully predicted by computer modelling (James and Cowe 1996). In cells, proteins could shield the target from interactions with a ribozyme molecule or they could facilitate the binding of a ribozyme to its target. In vitro experiments have shown that proteins, such as single-strand binding proteins, can enhance the catalytic effect of ribozymes by facilitating binding of the ribozyme to the target as well as product dissociation (Heidenreich et al. 1995; Tsuchihashi et al. 1993).

The Suitability of HIV as a Target for Gene Inhibition Therapy

The principal cellular hosts for HIV in vivo are cells of the macrophage lineage and CD4+ lymphocytes. The growing understanding of the rapid kinetics of infected cell turnover in vivo and the significance of the macrophage in pathogenesis (Embretson et al. 1993; Gartner and Popovic 1990; Lafeuillade et al. 1993; Macatonia et al. 1990; Pantaleo et al. 1991; Saksela et al. 1993; Watkins et al. 1990; Wei et al. 1995) provide hope for the use of gene therapy in the treatment of lymphocytes but discourage us from thinking that this will cure the disease. Although the precursors to macrophages (blood monocytes) and memory T cells are present in the circulation, and so amenable to ex vivo manipulation, many of their differentiated progeny are not. Both lineages are ultimately derived from CD34+ haemopoietic stem cells, which are a very tiny proportion of the normal haemopoietic tissue. Few of members of these populations are engaged in cell division at any one time and this, together with their expression of low levels of receptor for conventional retroviral vectors, makes them relatively refractory to transduction. In addition, the manipulation of stem cells in vitro tends to erode their pluripotency (Plavec et al. 1996). A number of methodological approaches are being used in an attempt to overcome these problems (see Fruehauf et al., this volume). Although some are essentially incremental improvements in standard techniques (Bahner et al. 1996; Leavitt et al. 1996), more radical approaches, such as the use of alternative oncovirus envelope glycoproteins (Baum et al. 1996), lentiviruses, such as HIV itself, as vectors for non-mitotic leukocytes (Haubrich et al. 1995; Naldini et al. 1996), or a combination of an HIV core in a *Vesiculovirus* envelope (Akkina et al. 1996), promise to bring significant improvements.

Sequence Variation in HIV

One of the greatest challenges to HIV gene therapy is the propensity for the virus to adapt by sequence variation to any therapeutic selection pressure. Clearly, ribozymes and antisense RNAs, which are sequence selective, are as liable as any therapeutic to this problem. One disadvantage of long antisense arm ribozymes is that they might become less sequence specific, cleaving poorly matched substrate RNAs (Herschlag 1991; Hertel et al. 1996). However, it turns out that they remain non-inhibitory to RNAs that lack extensive complementarity near the cleavage site but retain a substantial degree of inhibition against divergent strains. For example, when we challenge cells expressing the HIV-1_{IIIB}-*tat*-directed ribozyme $496_{33:33}$ with HIV-1 strains MN, SF2 and RF (which have 3, 5 and 5 mismatches, respectively, within the 66-nt region of complementarity), we retain over 90% inhibition of replication on days 7–10 post-challenge. In other pre-clinical assessments of anti-HIV ribozymes, conserved target sites have been chosen and shown to protect primary lymphocytes and CD34-derived macrophages from the effects of HIV replication (Lun Quan et al. 1995; Vandendriessche et al. 1995; Wong-Staal 1995).

The Clinical Trials for AIDS Gene Therapy

Apart from the vector system and the particular inhibitory constructs under study, the proposed gene therapy trials differ in the choice they make concerning two issues.

1) *CD34+ Stem Cells or Peripheral Blood Lymphocytes?* The former are much more difficult to work with, being hard to transduce and prone to unwanted differentiation. However the latter can only give rise to other lymphocytes, with the potential problem of clonal bias, and so neither macrophages nor other monocyte-derived cells will be protected. It is likely that any successful protocol will need to target both cell types in order to provide both immediate and long-term responses.
2) *Syngeneic or Autologous Cells?* The use of syngeneic donor cells, usually from identical twins with discordant HIV status, has the advantage that the donor can spare sufficient healthy cells and the in vitro manipulations will not amplify infectious virus. The latter have the advantage of being a reasonable model for the usual clinical situation and of affording a much greater population of study patients.

A "typical" phase I/II trial will have the following features:

1. Small number of discordant twins selected
2. Apheresis, peripheral blood mononuclear cells cut, CD4 enrichment
3. OK T4 stimulation
4. Enhancing culture conditions used: phosphate depletion, source of serum, cytokines, etc.
5. Enhancing transduction conditions used: temperature, centrifugation, protamine sulphate, etc.
6. Up to five rounds of transduction
7. More than one inhibitory gene, each with a distinct mechanism of action
8. A selectable marker present in the vector, in spite of the possibility of immunological rejection
9. Co-infusion of marked control and "protected" cells
10. Less than 2 weeks from apheresis to reinfusion
11. Up to 4 repeat infusions depending on the monitored indicators
12. Multiple indicators of recipients' health status:
    - Frequency of marked lymphocytes
    - Relative frequency of marked control and "protected" lymphocytes
    - Absence of replication-competent retrovirus
    - CD4:CD8 ratio
    - Plasma viraemia
    - p24 antigen
    - DTH-responses.

In the stalled trial sponsored by the University of California, San Diego and Immusol, 12 patients are expected to be treated with retroviral vectors encoding a pair of hairpin ribozymes expressed on the antisense strand from a tRNA promoter.

In the Morgan and Walker trial (Morgan and Walker 1996), the PBLs of discordant twin pairs will be transduced with retroviral vectors expressing both an antisense against trans-activation response element and the RevM10 trans-dominant construct. The aim of the study will be to determine the safety of the procedure and the longevity of the transduced cells.

In the Ribozyme Therapeutics Inc. trial, which has exemption from regulatory approval and is expecting FDA approval "very shortly", retroviral vectors will express two hammerhead ribozymes (against *tat* and *tat/rev*) in full-length transcripts. In pre-clinical experiments on G-CSF-elicited peripheral CD34+ cell-derived macrophages, these vectors have given up to 5-log infectivity reduction. In the clinical protocol, ten patients will be treated using freshly transduced, autologous, G-CSF-elicited CD34+ cells (both transduced with control, marker retrovirus and ribozyme-encoding virus).

In the Gene Shears trials, the first phase, which was due to begin in Australia in the third quarter of 1996; the CD4+ peripheral lymphocytes of the uninfected member of five pairs of discordant twins will be transduced with marker and hammerhead ribozyme-encoding retroviruses and reinfused into the HIV member of the pair. The trial will aim to test the longevity of the transduced cells in vivo and the safety of the procedure. A second trial is planned, to take place in the USA, using CD34+ haemopoietic stem cells.

Stop! Go! Stop!

At the time of writing, it could not be established that the ribozyme-based trials, which have been imminent for many months, had actually started. It is unclear why there are continued delays. We are aware of some disappointing laboratory results but it is conceivable that the apparent success of the conventional triple antiretroviral therapy has caused some patients to withdraw from study. Timing, in science as in comedy, is everything.

Acknowledgments. I am very grateful to Geoff Symons and John Rossi for disclosure of information about the Gene Shears and RPI trials, respectively.

References

Akkina RK, Walton RM, Meng Liang C, Li QX, Planelles V, Chen ISY (1996) High-efficiency gene transfer into CD34+ cells with a human immunodeficiency virus type 1-based retroviral vector pseudotyped with vesicular stimulatitis virus envelope glycoprotein G. J Virol 70:2581–2585

Bahner I, Kearns K, Hao QL, Smogorzewska EM, Kohn DB (1996) Transduction of human CD34+ hematopoietic progenitor cells by a retroviral vector expressing an RRE decoy inhibits human immunodeficiency virus type 1 replication in myelomonocytic cells produced in long-term culture. J Virol 70:4352–4360

Baum C, Eckert HG, Stockschlager M, Just U, Hegewisch-Becker S, Hildinger M, Uhde A, John J, Ostertag W (1996) Improved retroviral vectors for hematopoietic stem cell protection and in vivo selection. J Hematother 5:323–329

Bertrand E, Pictet R, Grange T (1994) Can hammerhead ribozymes be efficient tools to inactivate gene function? Nucleic Acids Res 22:293–300

Chen CJ, Banerjea AC, Harmison GG, Haglund K, Schubert M (1992) Multitarget-ribozyme directed to cleave at up to nine highly conserved HIV-1 env RNA regions inhibits HIV-1 replication-potential effectiveness against most presently sequenced HIV-1 isolates. Nucleic Acids Res 20:4581–4589

Cole-Strauss A, Yoon K, Xiang Y, Byrne BC, Rice MC, Gryn J, Holloman WK, Kmiec EB (1996) Correction of the mutation responsible for sickle cell anemia by an RNA-DNA oligonucleotide. Science 273:1386–1389

Crisell P, Thompson S, James W (1993) Inhibition of HIV-1 replication by ribozymes that show poor activity in vitro. Nucleic Acids Res 21:5251–5255

Dropulic B, Lin NH, Martin MA, Jeang KT (1992) Functional characterization of a U5 ribozyme: intracellular suppression of human immunodeficiency virus type 1 expression. J Virol 66:1432–1441

Embretson J, Zupancic M, Ribas JL, Burke A, Racz P, Tenner-Racz K, Haase AT (1993) Massive covert infection of helper T lymphocytes and macrophages by HIV during the incubation period of AIDS. Nature 362:359–362

Fedor MJ, Uhlenbeck OC (1990) Substrate sequence effects of 'hammerhead' RNA catalytic efficiency. Proc Natl Acad Sci USA 87:1668–1672

Gartner S, Popovic M (1990) Macrophage tropism of HIV-1. AIDS Res Hum Retroviruses 6:1017–1021

Goodchild J, Kohli V (1991) Ribozymes that cleave an RNA sequence from human immunodeficiency virus: the effect of flanking sequence on rate. Arch Biochem Biophys 284:386–391

Hampel A, Tritz R (1989) RNA catalytic properties of the minimum (-)sTRSV sequence. Biochemistry 28:4929–4933

Haseloff J, Gerlach W (1988) Simple RNA enzymes with new and highly specific endoribonuclease activities. Nature 334:585–591

Haubrich R, McCutchan JA, Holdredge R, Heiner L, Merritt J, Merchant B (1995) An open label, phase I/II clinical trial to evaluate the safety and biological activity of HIV-IT (V) (HIV-1 (IIIB)(env/rev) retroviral vector) in HIV-1-infected subjects. Hum Gene Ther 6:941–955

Heidenreich O, Kang SH, Brown DA, Xu X, Swiderski P, Rossi JJ, Eckstein F, Nerenberg M (1995) Ribozyme-mediated RNA degradation in nuclei suspension. Nucleic Acids Res 23:2223–2228

Herschlag D (1991) Implications of ribozyme kinetics for targeting the cleavage of specific RNA molecules in vivo: more isn't always better. Proc Natl Acad Sci USA 88:6921–6925

Hertel KJ, Herschlag D, Uhlenbeck OC (1994) A kinetic and thermodynamic framework for the hammerhead ribozyme reaction. Biochemistry 33:3374–3385

Hertel KJ, Herschlag D, Uhlenbeck OC (1996) Specificity of hammerhead rhibozyme cleavage. EMBO J 15:3751–3757

Homann M, Tzortzakaki S, Rittner K; Sczakiel G, Tabler M (1993) Incorporation of the catalytic domain of a hammerhead ribozyme into antisense RNA enhances its inhibitory effect on the replication of human immunodeficiency virus type 1. Nucleic Acids Res 2809–2814

James W, Cowe E (1996) Computational approaches to the identification of ribozyme target sites. In: Turner P (ed) Methods in molecular biology. Humana, Totowa (in press)

Laufeillade A, Tamalet C, Pellegrino P, Tourres C, Yahi N, Vignoli C, Quilichini R, De MP (1993) High viral burden in lymph nodes during early stages of HIV-1 infection (1). AIDS 7:1527–1528

Leavitt MC, Yu M, Wong-Staal F, Looney DJ (1996) Ex vivo transduction and expansion of CD4+ lymphocytes from HIV+ donors: prelude to a ribozyme gene therapy trial. Gene Ther 3:599–606

Lo KM, Biasolo MA, Dehni G, Palu G, Haseltine WA (1992) Inhibition of replication of HIV-1 by retroviral vectors expressing tat-antisense and anti-tat ribozyme RNA. Virology 190:176–183

Lun Quan S, Pyati J, Smythe J, Wang L, Macpherson J, Gerlach W, Symonds G (1995) Resistance to human immunodeficiency virus type 1 infection conferred by transduction of human peripheral blood lymphocytes with ribozyme, antisense, or polymeric trans-activation response element constructs. Proc Natl Acad Sci USA 92:7272–7276

Macatonia SE, Lau R, Patterson S, Pinching AJ, Knight SC (1990) Dendritic cell infection, depletion and dysfunction in HIV-infected individuals. Immunology 71:38–45

Morgan R, Walker R (1996) Gene therapy for AIDS using retroviral mediated gene transfer to deliver HIV-1 antisense TAR and transdominant Rev protein genes to syngeneic lymphocytes in HIV-1 infected identical twins. Hum Gene Ther 7:1281–1306

Naldini L, Blomer U, Gallay P, Ory D, Mulligan R, Gage FH, Verma IM, Trono D (1996) In vivo gene delivery and stable transduction of nondividing cells by a lentiviral vector. Science 272:263–267

Ojwang JO, Hampel A, Looney DJ, Wong-Staal F, Rappaport J (1992) Inhibition of human immunodeficiency virus type 1 expression by a hairpin ribozyme. Proc Natl Acad USA 89:10802–10806

Pantaleo G, Graziosi C, Butini L, Pizzo PA, Schnittman SM, Kotler DP, Fauci AS (1991) Lymphoid organs function as major reservoirs for human immunodeficiency virus. Proc Natl Acad Sci USA 88:9838–9842

Perriman R, Delves A, Gerlach WL (1992) Extended target-site specificity for a hammerhead ribozyme. Gene 113:157–163

Plavec I, Voytovich A, Moss K, Webster D, Hanley MB, Escaich S, Ho KE, Bohnlein E, DiGiusto DL (1996) Sustained retroviral gene marking and expression in lymphoid and myeloid cells derived from transduced hematopoietic progenitor cells. Gene Ther 3:717–724

Rhodes A, James W (1990) Inhibition of human immunodeficiency virus replication in cell culture by endogenously synthesized antisense RNA. J Gen Virol 71:1965–1974

Rhodes A, James W (1991) Inhibition of heterologous strains of HIV by antisense RNA [see comments]. AIDS 5:145–151

Saksela K, Muchmore E, Girard M, Fultz P, Baltimore D (1993) High viral load in lymph nodes and latent human immunodeficiency virus (HIV) in peripheral blood cells of HIV-1-infected chimpanzees. J Virol 67:7423–7427

Sarver N, Cantin EM, Chang PS, Zaia JA, Ladne PA, Stephens DA, Rossi JJ (1990) Ribozymes as potential anti-HIV-1 therapeutic agents. Science 247:1222–1225

Sczakiel G, Pawlita M, Kleinheinz A (1990) Specific inhibition of human immunodeficiency virus type 1 replication by RNA transcribed in sense and antisense orientation from the 5′-leader/gap region. Biochem Biophys Res Commun 169:643–651

Tabler M, Tsagris M (1991) Catalytic antisense RNAs produced by incorporating ribozyme cassettes into cDNA. Gene 108:175–183

Tabler M, Homann M, Tzortzakaki S, Sczakiel G (1994) A three-nucleotide helix I is sufficient for full activity of a hammerhead ribozyme: advantages of an asymmetric design. Nucleic Acids Res 22:3958–3965

Tsuchihashi Z, Khosla M, Herschlag D (1993) Protein enhancement of hammerhead ribozyme catalysis. Science 262:99–101

Uhlenbeck OC (1987) A small catalytic oligoribonucleotide. Nature 328:596–600

Vandendriessche T, Chuah MKL, Chiang L, Chang HK, Ensoli B, Morgan RA (1995) Inhibition of clinical human immunodeficiency virus (HIV) type 1 isolates in primary CD4+ T lymphocytes by retroviral vectors expressing anti-HIV genes. J Virol 69:4045–4052

Watkins BA, Dorn HH, Kelly WB, Armstrong RC, Potts BJ, Michaels F, Kufta CV, Dubois DM (1990) Specific tropism of HIV-1 for microglial cells in primary human brain cultures. Science 249:549–553

Wei X, Ghosh S, Taylor M, Johnson V, Emini E, Deutsch P, Lifson J, Bonhoeffer S, Nowak M et al (1995) Viral dynamics in HIV-1 infection. Nature 373:117–122

Wong-Staal F (1995) Ribozyme gene therapy for HIV infection. Intracellular immunization of lymphocytes and CD34+ cells with an anti-HIV-1 ribozyme gene. Adv Drug Deliv Rev 17:363–368

Yoon K, Cole-Strauss A, Kmiec EB (1996) Targeted gene correction of episomal DNA in mammalian cells mediated by a chimeric RNA-DNA oligonucleotide. Proc Natl Acad Sci USA 93:2071–2076

Yu M, Ojwang J, Yamada O, Hampel A, Rapapport J, Looney D, Wong-Staal F (1993) A hairpin ribozyme inhibits expression of diverse strains of human immunodeficiency virus type 1. Proc Natl Acad Sci USA 90:6340–6344

Subject Index

MIX
Papier aus verantwortungsvollen Quellen
Paper from responsible sources
FSC® C105338

If you have any concerns about our products,
you can contact us on
ProductSafety@springernature.com

In case Publisher is established outside the EU,
the EU authorized representative is:
Springer Nature Customer Service Center GmbH
Europaplatz 3, 69115 Heidelberg, Germany

Printed by Libri Plureos GmbH
in Hamburg, Germany